Carcinogenesis: Recent Investigations

Papers by
Fred G. Bock, Judith G. Tasseron, Peter
J. Bryant et al.

MSS Information Corporation
655 Madison Avenue, New York, N.Y. 10021

Library of Congress Cataloging in Publication Data
Main entry under title:

Carcinogenesis: recent investigations.

  Includes bibliographical references.
  1. Carcinogenesis. I. Bock, Fred G.
RC268.5.C37   616.9'94'071   72-6311
ISBN 0-8422-7017-5

TABLE OF CONTENTS

CREDITS AND ACKNOWLEDGMENTS

Basrur, Parvathi K.; Anthony K. Sykes; and J. P. W. Gilman, "Changes in Mitochondrial Ultrastructure in Nickel Sulfide-Induced Rhabdomyosarcoma," *Cancer*, 1970, 25:1142—1152.

Bock, Fred G., "The Nature of Tumor-Promoting Agents in Tobacco Products," *Cancer Research*, 1968, 28:2363—2368.

Bock, Fred G.; Audrey Fjelde; Helen W. Fox; and Edmund Klein, "Tumor Promotion by 1-Fluoro-2,4-dinitrobenzene, a Potent Skin Sensitizer," *Cancer Research*, 1969, 29:179—182.

Bryant, Peter J.; and James H. Sang, "Physiological Genetics of Melanotic Tumors in *Drosophila melanogaster*. VI. The Tumorigenic Effects of Juvenile Hormone-Like Substances, " *Genetics*, 1969, 62:321—336.

Chen, T. T.; and Charles Heidelberger, "Quantitative Studies on the Malignant Transformation of Mouse Prostate Cells by Carcinogenic Hydrocarbons *in Vitro*," *International Journal of Cancer*, 1969, 4:166—178.

Grunberger, Dezider; James H. Nelson; Charles R. Cantor; and I. Bernard Weinstein, "Coding and Conformational Properties of Oligonucleotides Modified with the Carcinogen *N*-2-Acetylaminofluorene," *Proceedings of the National Academy of Sciences*, 1970, 66:488—494.

Krarup, Torben, "Oocyte Destruction and Ovarian Tumorigenesis after Direct Application of a Chemical Carcinogen (9:10-Dimethyl-1:2-Benzanthracene) to the Mouse Ovary," *International Journal of Cancer*, 1969, 4:61—75.

Lotlikar, Prabhakar, "Effects of 3-Methylcholanthrene Pretreatment of Microsomal Hydroxylation of 2-Acetamidofluorene by Various Rat Hepatomas," *Biochemistry Journal*, 1970, 118:513—518.

Matsuyama, M.; and H. Suzuki, "Adrenal Tumours and Endocrine Lesions Induced in Syrian Hamsters by Urethane Injected during Suckling Period," *The British Journal of Cancer*, 1970, 24:312—318.

Pound, A. W., "The Influence of Preliminary Irritation by Acetic Acid or Croton Oil on Skin Tumour Production in Mice after a Single Application of Dimethylbenzanthracene, Benzopyrene, or Dibenzanthracene," *The British Journal of Cancer*, 1968, 22:533—544.

Sato, Kei; Tadayuki Saito; and Makoto Enomoto, "Development of Sarcomas in Mice at Site of Injection with a New Carcinogen, Monoacetyl Derivative of 4-Hydroxyaminoquinoline," *The Japanese Journal of Experimental Medicine*, 1970, 40:475–478.

Sato, Kiyomi; Toshio Kuroki; and Haruo Sato, "Respiration and Glycolysis of Cells Transformed with 4-Nitroquinoline-1-Oxide and Its Derivative (34776)," *Proceedings of the Society for Experimental Biology and Medicine*, 1970, 134:281–283.

Shimkin, M. B.; T. Sasaki; M. McDonough; R. Baserga; D. Thatcher; and R. Wieder, "Relation of Thymidine Index to Pulmonary Tumor Response in Mice Receiving Urethan and Other Carcinogens," *Cancer Research*, 1969, 29:994–998.

Shisa, Hayase, "Studies on the Mechanism of 7,12-Dimethylbenz[a]anthracene Leukemogenesis in Mice. II. The Role of Thymus in DMBA Leukemogenesis," *Mie Medical Journal*, 1969, 19:101–109.

Sugimoto, Tsutomu; and Hiroshi Terayama, "Studies on Carcinogen-Binding Proteins. I. Isolation and Characterization of Aminoazo Dye-Bound Protein after Administration of a Single Large Dose of 3-Methyl-4-Dimethylaminoazobenzene to Rats," *Biochimica et Biophysica Acta*, 1970, 214:533–544.

Tasseron, Judith G.; Heino Diringer; Nechama Frohwirth; S. S. Mirvish; and Charles Heidelberger, "Partial Purification of Soluble Protein from Mouse Skin to which Carcinogenic Hydrocarbons Are Specifically Bound," *Biochemistry*, 1970, 9:1636–1644.

Wynder, Ernest L.; and Dietrich Hoffmann, "A Study of Tobacco Carcinogenesis X. Tumor Promoting Activity," *Cancer*, 1969, 24:289–301.

Carcinogenic Effects of Specific Compounds

ADRENAL TUMOURS AND ENDOCRINE LESIONS INDUCED IN SYRIAN HAMSTERS BY URETHANE INJECTED DURING SUCKLING PERIOD

M. MATSUYAMA AND H. SUZUKI

URETHANE has been found to be a multipotential carcinogen in several strains of mice. Tumours of various organs including the lung, liver, ovary, thymus, lymph node, Harderian gland and others, are induced (Tannenbaum and Silverstone, 1958; Della Porta et al., 1967; Vesselinovitch and Mihailovich, 1967; Matsuyama and Suzuki, 1968). Urethane also has a broad spectrum of action in rats inducing pulmonary adenomas, hepatomas, brain tumours, mammary fibroadenomas, and uterine sarcomas (Jaffe, 1947; Tannenbaum et al., 1962; Vesselinovitch and Mihailovich, 1968a and b). The target organs for this carcinogen in Syrian hamsters differ from those in mice and rats. Melanotic tumours of the skin and papillomas of the forestomach are induced when this chemical is administered to hamsters in the drinking water (Pietra and Shubik, 1960; Toth, Tomatis and Shubik, 1961).

This report describes the effects of urethane given by subcutaneous injection to suckling Syrian golden hamsters.

MATERIALS AND METHODS

Experimental animals.—Syrian golden hamsters, obtained from Dr. H. Uno, Department of Pathology, Nagoya University, Nagoya, and bred in our laboratory by sister-to-brother mating since 1965, were used. The colony originally came from the Cancer Research Institute, New England Deaconess Hospital, Boston, to the National Institute of Health, Tokyo, in 1959, and then to Dr. Uno in 1964.

Experimental procedure.—Animals from seven litters were given, in the interscapular region, 6-weekly subcutaneous injections of a 10% saline solution of urethane (E. Merck, Darmstadt) at a dose of 1 mg./g. of body weight. The injections were started at 7 days of age. Another ten litters that received no treatment served as controls. Following treatment the animals were kept separate from their mothers for about 3 hours to avoid maternal cannibalism. The litters were weaned and separated by sex at 6 weeks of age. They were housed in aluminium cages with sawdust bedding and were given CMF diet (Oriental Yeast, Tokyo) and water *ad libitum*.

The hamsters injected with urethane were permitted to live out their life span. Animals found in a semi-comatose condition were killed. The experiment was terminated at the end of 124 weeks, because the last female hamster injected with urethane died on the 728th day and the last male died on the 864th day. The surviving controls were killed at 104 weeks for females and 124 weeks for males. Complete necropsies were performed on all animals killed or found dead. The adrenals, thyroid gland, pituitary, ovaries, testes, pancreas, lungs, liver, spleen, Harderian glands, and other organs which showed grossly visible tumours were fixed in 10% formalin solution, sectioned and stained with haematoxylin and eosin. For electron microscopy, other areas of the pancreas were fixed in 3% glutaraldehyde buffered with 0·1 M phosphate for 3 hours and postfixed in 2% osmium tetroxide buffered with 0·1 M phosphate for 3 hours. The tissue blocks were dehydrated in graded ethanols, and then embedded in Epon 812. Ultrathin sections were cut on an LKB ultratome and stained with uranyl acetate and lead (Sato, 1968). Grids were studied with an Hitachi HU-11B electron microscope. Routine determinations of blood sugar were performed by using Dextrostix (Ames Japan, Tokyo).

RESULTS

The survival, localization and frequency of tumours and lesions observed in the experimental and control groups are shown in Table I. The 6-weekly injections of urethane significantly reduced the survival. Most of the animals, which were injected with urethane and survived more than 52 weeks, became semi-comatose for 2–6 days before death, and were severely emaciated. They usually showed severe hypoglycaemia with a blood glucose below 40 mg./ml. At autopsy a small to moderate volume of clear ascitic fluid was present and nodules of histiocytosis in atrophic spleens were noted in many of these animals.

Adrenal hyperplasia.—Most of the hamsters injected with urethane developed adrenal hyperplasia whereas this lesion was observed in only a few of the control animals (Table I). The lesion was first found in an injected, female hamster killed at 377 days after birth. In the control animals this was observed at 510 postnatal days. The surface of the adrenals was either translucent and normal appearing or characterized by the presence of whitish yellow pin-point spots. Histologically there were three types of nodular hyperplasia, including small spindle-shaped cells, densely packed medium-sized cells, or large eosinophilic granular cells. The nodular hyperplasia was bilateral and multicentric. Thus, the same adrenal frequently contained several nodules which varied in size and showed different cell types. These lesions seemed to originate usually from the zona glomerulosa and compressed the zona fasciculata and the zona reticularis (Fig. 1). Some of them showed marked displacement of the medulla (Fig. 2). In these cases a few mitotic figures were seen and a capsule bordering these lesions was lacking.

Adrenal tumours.—Macroscopical adrenal cortical tumours were produced in 8 hamsters (6 females and 2 males) injected with urethane (Table I). The first tumour was found in a female hamster killed at 492 days after birth. In the

9

TABLE I.—*Induction of Tumours and Other Lesions in Hamsters Injected with Urethane During Suckling Period*

Treatment	Sex	Survival time (weeks)	Adrenal hyperplasia No. of animals	(%*)	Adrenal tumours No. of animals	(%*)	β-cell proliferation in pancreatic islet No. of animals	(%*)	Other lesions
Urethane†	F	0 6 26 52 78 104 30 26 25 20 12 0	19	(95)	6	(30)	17	(85)	3 adenomatous hyperplasia of thyroid 19 spleen nodules of histiocytosis. 3 melanomas of skin and eyelids 4 papillomas of forestomach 3 haemangiomas of liver 1 adenocarcinoma of exocrine pancreas 2 cysts of liver
	M	11 9 9 8 6 4	7	(88)	2	(25)	7	(75)	1 β-cell tumour of pancreatic islet 7 spleen nodules of histiocytosis 1 haemangioma of liver 2 cysts of liver
None	F	31 27 26 25 21 12‡	9	(36)	0	(—)	2	(8)	2 cysts of liver 1 papilloma of forestomach
	M	34 31 30 26 20‡	9	(30)	0	(—)	3	(10)	1 adenomatous hyperplasia of thyroid 3 cysts of liver

* Percentages are given on survivors at 52 weeks after birth.
† Each animal was given 6-weekly subcutaneous injections at a dose of 1 mg./g. of body weight, starting at 7 days of age.
‡ These were killed 104th week for the females and in 124th week for the males, and the experiment was terminated.

males the tumour developed later (788 and 815 days after birth). Two of the tumours were yellow, soft and bean-size (Fig. 3). Histologically narrow rims of nontumourous cortical tissue, which contained hyperplastic nodules of different types, surrounded the tumours. The border of the tumours was well defined, but no capsule was evident. The tumours consisted of medium sized, densely packed cells with eosinophilic cytoplasm, showing a trabecular pattern (Fig. 4). A few mitotic cells were noted. Four others were yellow-white, soft, and finger-tip sized tumours. No cortical tissue was observed around the tumour masses, except cysts. The tumours consisted of two or three types of cells; small spindle-shaped cells, medium sized densely packed cells, and/or large granular cells, with intermingled areas of these cell types (Fig. 5 and 6). Mitotic cells were not frequent. There was no infiltration or metastases in other organs. The tumours were unilateral, and the contralateral glands were slightly atrophic, weighing 5–10 mg. The remaining two tumours in the female hamsters were of thumb size and had infiltrations and/or metastases in the kidney, liver, periportal- and perigastric lymph nodes, and lungs (Fig. 7). The tumours consisted of large polygonal and pleomorphic cells (Fig. 8), containing large areas of coagulation necrosis and haemorrhage.

Other endocrine lesions.—The majority of hamsters injected with urethane showed proliferation of densely packed cells in the centre of the pancreatic islets (Table I and Fig. 9). This β-cell proliferation was first noticed in a female hamster killed at 425 days after birth. In the control animals this was found only in the hamsters killed at the end of the experiment, 104 weeks after birth for the females and 124 weeks for the males. These proliferating cells were oval with vesicular nuclei and narrow, eosinophilic-granular cytoplasm, in which a few but definite

---

EXPLANATION OF PLATES

Fig. 1.—Subcapsular nodular hyperplasia of granular cell type compresses the zona fasciculata. H. and E.   × 59.

Fig. 2.—Nodular hyperplasia of compact cell type replaces the zona fasciculata and the zona reticularis, and invades into the medulla. H. and E.   × 59.

Fig. 3.—Bean sized tumour in the left adrenal gland, with area of subcapsular bleeding. Two-thirds was removed for transplantation and for electron microscopy. Atrophy of right adrenal (lower). × 2·4.

Fig. 4.—Same hamster shown in Fig. 3. Tumour of medium sized compact cell type, showing trabecular pattern. H. and E.   × 445.

Fig. 5.—Area of adrenal tumour consisting of spindle cells. H. and E.   × 445.

Fig. 6.—Same hamster shown in Fig. 5. Another area of the tumour consisting of large granular cells, showing large discrete nucleoli. H. and E.   × 445.

Fig. 7.—Tumour in the right adrenal gland with the infiltration into the right kidney and liver. Multiple metastatic nodules in the lungs (upper) and periportal- and perigastric-lymph nodes (lower right) are also shown. × 1·1.

Fig. 8.—Same hamster shown in Fig. 7. Tumour cells are large and pleomorphic, with many mitotic figures. H. and E.   × 445.

Fig. 9.—Same hamster shown in Fig. 7 and 8. In the centre of the islet proliferation of small, eosinophilic stained cells are shown. H. and E.   × 289.

Fig. 10.—Electron micrograph taken from a pancreatic islet of a female hamster injected with urethane. A β-cell with narrow cytoplasm containing a few β-cell granules (arrows) is shown. Stained with uranyl acetate and lead. × 7320.

Fig. 11.—Same hamster shown in Fig. 3 and 4. Beta-cell tumour of the pancreatic islet consisting of cells which have large vesicular nuclei and irregular shaped, slightly eosinophilic cytoplasm, showing mosaic pattern and intimate relationship with capillaries. H. and E. × 445.

Fig. 12.—Same hamster shown in Fig. 7, 8, and 9. Adenomatous hyperplasia of the thyroid. H. and E.   × 67.

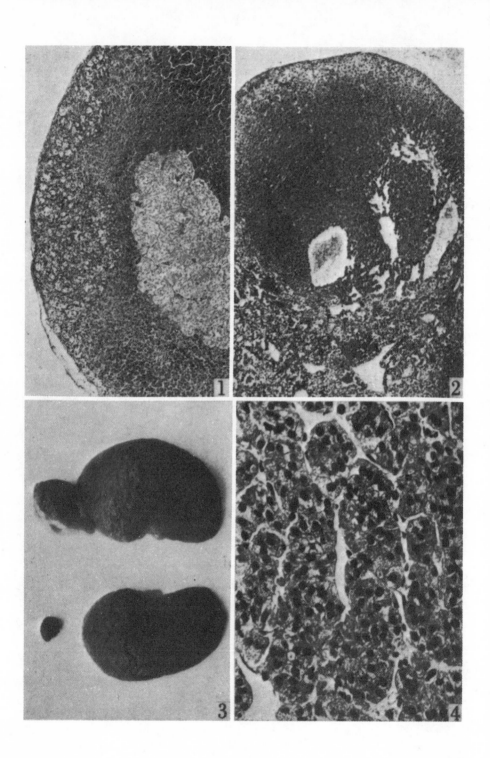

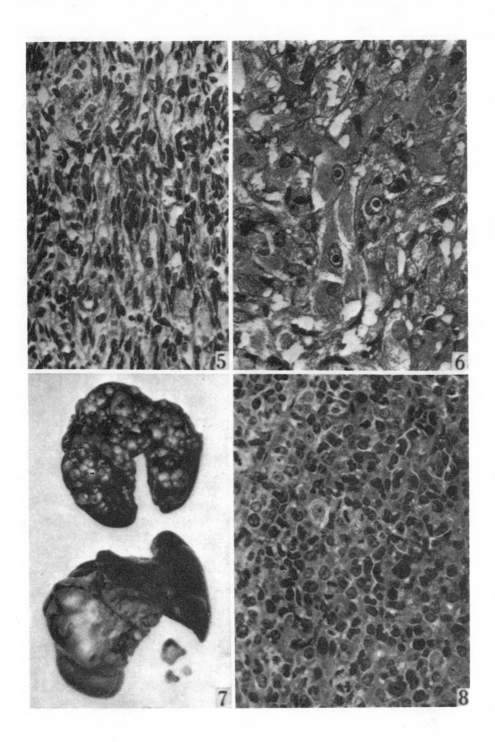

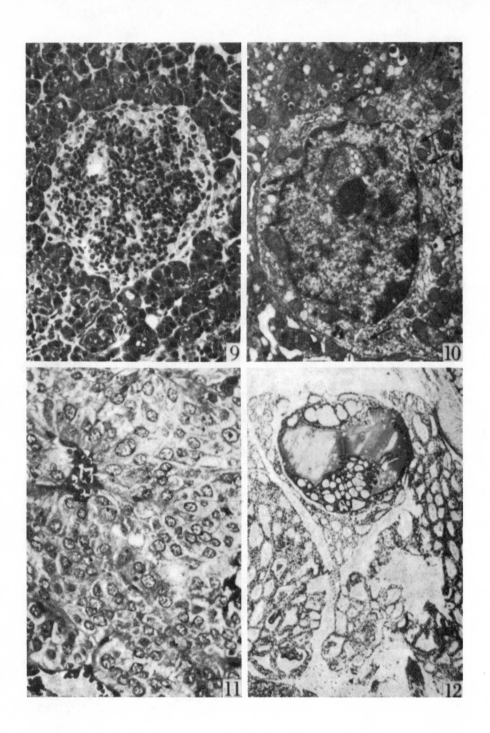

14

β-cell granules were found submicroscopically (Fig. 10). A β-cell tumour was found in a male hamster injected with urethane, age 788 days (Table I). The tumour, which was in the deeper area of the pancreas, was noticed by red colour of a blood lake contained in the mass. It was ovoid, of rice size, and surrounded by a thick capsule. The tumour cells were large and stained slightly eosinophilic, and had an intimate relationship to abundant capillaries (Fig. 11). A number of dark stained and pyknotic cells was scattered among the clear large cells, but mitoses were seldom identified. Submicroscopically it was diagnosed as a β-cell tumour of the pancreatic islet.

Adenomatous hyperplasia of the thyroid gland was also found in three female hamsters injected with urethane and in one male control animal (Table I and Fig. 12). The pituitaries, ovaries, and testes were severely atrophic in the animals injected with urethane. In addition to the endocrine lesions, other types of lesions were also found in a few treated and control hamsters (Table I).

DISCUSSION

Neonatal injection of 150 μg. of urethane failed to induce tumours in Syrian golden hamsters (Walters, Roe and Levene, 1967). This was probably because the dose, which may correspond to 0·06–0·07 mg./g. of body weight, was too low. The administration of urethane in the drinking water (0·2%) to 8- to 10-week-old hamsters gave rise to melanotic tumours of the skin in a moderate percentage (Pietra and Shubik, 1960). Using larger doses (0·2 and 0·4%) and younger animals, 5- to 7-weeks old, Toth, Tomatis and Shubik (1961) induced melanotic tumours in a higher percentage. Papillomas and carcinomas of the forestomach, malignant lymphomas, and liver tumours also developed. The present experiment, using suckling hamsters and subcutaneous injections of still larger doses, succeeded in producing endocrine lesions besides melanotic tumours. This may be due to the age of the animals used. Such a change in the target organs of a carcinogen because of difference in age of animals has been demonstrated in the types of mouse tumours induced by 7,12-dimethylbenz(a)anthracene (DMBA), dimethylnitrosamine, and urethane (Pietra, Rappaport, and Shubik, 1961; Toth Rappaport, and Shubik, 1963; Terracini et al., 1966; Della Porta et al., 1967; Vesselinovitch and Mihailovich, 1967).

Spontaneous adrenal cortical tumours in hamsters are not infrequent and 4 adenomas were found in 51 untreated animals (Kirkman, 1950). However, adrenal tumours in hamsters induced by carcinogens have rarely been reported in the literature. Kirkman and Robbins (1956) found 35 adrenal cortical tumours, one a carcinoma, among 64 male and female hamsters that lived with subcutaneously implanted testosterone pellets for 608–950 days. Toth (1969) recently reported that 10 adrenal tumours were found in 60 young adult hamsters injected intravenously with 3 mg. of DMBA. In the present experiment 8 adrenal tumours, 2 with metastases, were found in 28 hamsters injected with urethane. Multiple areas of nodular hyperplasia were also present in the adrenal cortex. These two types of adrenal lesions had three different histological patterns; small spindle cell type, medium sized compact cell type and large granular cell type. It was therefore difficult to establish specific criteria for the histological diagnosis of hyperplasia, adenoma and carcinoma. Thus a simple biological classification was adopted, determined by the gross appearance of tumours and

15

the presence of metastases. It is noteworthy that the tumours are usually preceded by hyperplastic nodules.

Using a particular strain of mice (CE), Woolley and Little (1945) reported that neonatal ovariectomy gave rise to a high percentage of unusual, localized groups of "type A" or "type B" cells in the adrenal cortex and of the adrenal tumours. Among their 21 cases the tumours were bilateral in 11, differing sharply from the results of the present experiment in which all 8 tumours were unilateral and the contralateral glands were atrophic. In mice total-body neutron irradiation and treatment with DMBA also induced nonmetastasizing tumours of the adrenal cortex in 2·7–30% (Haran-Ghera et al., 1959; Mody, 1969).

Spontaneous islet cell tumours of the pancreas are rare in rodents (Rowlatt, 1967). Three adenomas and one adenocarcinoma of the islets were found in 7200 autopsied golden hamsters. Some were in control animals and the other animals had been subjected to a wide variety of surgical and/or other experimental treatments (Kirkman, 1962). Fortner (1957, 1961) reported six islet cell tumours in 181 hamsters. In the present study a β-cell tumour of the pancreatic islet was found in a male hamster injected with urethane. Thus it is difficult to decide whether the tumour was spontaneous, accelerated or induced. However, generalized hyperplasia of compact β-cells in the islets was noted in the majority of the treated animals.

Multiple tumours of endocrine glands, particularly of the pituitary, parathyroids, and adrenal glands, are known to be associated with islet cell tumours in man (Frantz, 1959). Berdjis (1960, 1963a, b) has reported that multiple endocrine tumours can be induced in the rat by whole or partial body irradiation. Gilbert and Gillman (1958) found a high incidence of endocrine tumours in different combinations in 1342 rats, but felt that there was no evidence that neoplastic change in one gland influenced the occurrence of neoplasia in another. However, the coexistence of nodular hyperplasia and tumours of the adrenal cortex and hyperplasia of the pancreatic islet, in the majority of the animals in the present study, is suggestive of severe hormonal disorders. Since hamsters bearing a transplantable adrenal cortical tumour, derived from a tumour induced in the present experiment, have shown the same type of hyperplasia in the pancreatic islet (Matsuyama and Suzuki, unpublished), it is reasonable to assume that the induction of the lesions in the pancreatic islet in the hamsters may be influenced by the presence of the adrenal lesions.

We are grateful to Professors T. Nagayo and Y. Nishizuka of this Institute, Dr. K. McD. Herrold, National Cancer Institute, Bethesda, and Professor S. Morii, Kansai Medical School, for their advice. One of us (M.M.) thanks the Lady Tata Memorial Trust for support by a Lady Tata Memorial Fellowship.

REFERENCES

BERDJIS, C. C.—(1960) Oncologia, Basel, 13, 441.—(1963a) Exp. molec. Path., 2, 157.—(1963b) Oncologia, Basel, 16, 81.
DELLA PORTA, G., CAPITANO, J., PARMI, L. AND COLNAGHI, M. I.—(1967) Tumori, 53, 81.
FORTNER, J. G.—(1957) Cancer, N.Y., 10, 1153.—(1961) Cancer Res., 21, 1491.
FRANTZ, V. K.—(1959) 'Tumors of the Pancreas. Atlas of Tumor Pathology'. Section 7, fasc. 27 and 28. Washington, D.C. (Armed Forces Institute of Pathology).

GILBERT, C. AND GILLMAN, J.—(1958) *S. Afr. J. med. Sci.*, **23**, 257.

HARAN-GHERA, N., FURTH, J., BUFFETT, R. F. AND YOKORO, K.—(1959) *Cancer Res.*, **19**, 1181.

JAFFE, W. G.—(1947) *Cancer Res.*, **7**, 107.

KIRKMAN, H.—(1950) *Anat. Rec.*, **106**, 277.—(1962) *Stanford med. Bull.*, **20**, 163.

KIRKMAN, H. AND ROBBINS, M.—(1956) *Proc. Am. Ass. Cancer Res.*, **2**, 125.

MATSUYAMA, M. AND SUZUKI, H.—(1968) *Br. J. Cancer*, **22**, 527.

MODY, J. K.—(1969) *Cancer Res.*, **29**, 1254.

PIETRA, G., RAPPAPORT, H. AND SHUBIK, P.—(1961) *Cancer, N.Y.*, **14**, 308.

PIETRA, G. AND SHUBIK, P.—(1960) *J. natn. Cancer Inst.*, **25**, 627.

ROWALTT, U.—(1967) *Br. J. Cancer*, **21**, 82.

SATO, T.—(1968) *J. Electron Microscopy, Tokyo*, **17**, 158.

TANNENBAUM, A. AND SILVERSTONE, H.—(1958) *Cancer Res.*, **18**, 1225.

TANNENBAUM, A., VESSELINOVITCH, S. D., MALTONI, C. AND STRYZAK-MITCHELL, D.—(1962) *Cancer Res.*, **22**, 1363.

TERRACINI, B., PALESTRO, G., GIGLIARDI, M. R. AND MONTESANO, R.—(1966) *Br. J. Cancer*, **20**, 871.

TOTH, B.—(1969) *Cancer Res.*, **29**, 1476.

TOTH, B., RAPPAPORT, H. AND SHUBIK, P.—(1963) *J. natn. Cancer Inst.*, **30**, 723.

TOTH, B., TOMATIS, L. AND SHUBIK, P.—(1961) *Cancer Res.*, **21**, 1537.

VESSELINOVITCH, S. D. AND MIHAILOVICH, N.—(1967) *Cancer Res.*, **27**, 1422.—(1968a) *Cancer Res.*, **28**, 881.—(1968b) *Cancer Res.*, **28**, 888.

WALTERS, M. A., ROE, F. J. C. AND LEVENE, A.—(1967) *Br. J. Cancer*, **21**, 184.

WOOLLEY, G. W. AND LITTLE, C. C.—(1945) *Cancer Res.*, **5**, 193.

Relation of Thymidine Index to Pulmonary Tumor Response in Mice Receiving Urethan and Other Carcinogens

M. B. Shimkin, T. Sasaki, M. McDonough, R. Baserga, D. Thatcher, and R. Wieder

INTRODUCTION

A considerable body of literature has accumulated over the past 30 years on the subject of primary pulmonary tumors in mice as summarized in several reviews (17, 21). To the classical approaches of cancer biology, genetics, and histology, more recently have been added considerations of mathematical statistics (14) and of biochemistry (1).

Since neoplasms involve the production of new tissue, the relationship of DNA synthesis before and during the appearance of the gross neoplasm is of obvious importance. During the past two years, we have conducted several experiments

18

that provide data on DNA synthesis as measured by the incorporation of tritiated thymidine in mice exposed to several carcinogenic agents known to produce lung tumors. These are now reported.

EXPERIMENT 1

Materials and Methods

Two-month-old strain A/He male mice, weighing approximately 20 gm each, were administered single intraperitoneal injections of a 10% aqueous solution of ethyl carbamate (urethan), 1 mg/gm body weight.

Groups of 3 mice were injected subcutaneously with thymidine-methyl-^{3}H (6.7 c/mmole), 25 μc per animal, at intervals of 1 to 21 days following urethan.

The animals were killed by cervical dislocation 30 minutes after thymidine-^{3}H and the lungs removed and fixed in calcium-buffered formalin. Three mice that did not receive urethan were included as controls at Days 1 and 10.

Sections were autoradiographed as previously described (3), using Eastman Kodak NTB emulsion and an exposure time of 25 days. The developed autoradiographs were stained with hematoxylin and eosin. The fraction of labeled cells was determined by counting 3000 cells in each lung and is expressed here as the thymidine index (2).

Results

The results are given in Table 1. Within 24 hours there occurs a significant decrease in the thymidine index, presumably indicating inhibition of DNA synthesis. By 3 days there is recovery, and a rapid increase in the number of labeled alveolar cells, reaching a peak at 7 to 10 days that is at least 5-fold that of the control mice. At 21 days the number of labeled cells is still above that of the controls. At 21 days following this dose of urethan, microscopic pulmonary tumors can be identified (19); one such nodule was found in one section, and the number of labeled cells was 25 per 1000 or at the level of the peak of the general reaction observed 2 weeks earlier.

The depression at 1 day, and a 5-fold increase at 10 days, is also observed in the epithelial cells of the bronchi and bronchioles.

EXPERIMENT 2

Materials and Methods

Two-month-old strain A/He male mice, weighing ap-

19

proximately 20 gm each, were given single intraperitoneal injections on a per gram of body weight basis, of the following compounds and doses: (a) urethan, 1.0 mg; (b) urethan, 0.25 mg; (c) isopropyl carbamate, 1.0 mg; (d) methyl-bis-(β-chloroethyl)-amine hydrochloride (nitrogen mustard, HN2), 0.002 mg; and (e) 3-methylcholanthrene (MCA), 0.05 mg. Aqueous solutions were employed for all but MCA, which was dissolved in tricaprylin.

Table 1

| Days after urethan | No. of mice | Labeled cells/1000 cells | | | |
| | | Alveolar | | Bronchial | |
		Mean	Range	Mean	Range
0	9	6.7	5−9	1.3	1−2
1	3	2.5	1−4	0.5	0−1
3	3	6.2	4−10	1.3	0−3
7	3	29.5	25−36	5.0	4−6
10	3	26.0	11−36	6.0	1−8
14	3	12.7	7−28	3.3	2−5
21	3	9.8	7−14	2.0	1−3

Thymidine index of lung cells of strain A/He mice following a single intraperitoneal dose of urethan, 1 mg per gm body weight. Mice were killed 30 min after the injection of thymidine-^{3}H.

Following injection of the compounds, groups of 3 mice were injected subcutaneously with thymidine-^{3}H, at intervals of 1, 3, 5, 8, 14, and 21 days following injection of the carcinogens. Thirty minutes later they were killed, and the procedures outlined in Experiment 1 were followed.

Results

The results are given in Table 2. The initial decrease in the thymidine index, and a sharp increase at 8 days following the 1-mg-per-gm dose of urethan, closely replicates the findings of Experiment 1. However, with the smaller dose of 0.25 mg per gm, neither the initial inhibition, nor the sharp rebound are to be seen. Both dose levels of urethan produce pulmonary tumors in 100% of strain A/He mice within 20 weeks, and an average of 16 and 8 tumors per animal respectively can be

20

anticipated. Thus, the data suggest that the DNA suppression and subsequent enhancement are not directly related to carcinogenesis but, rather, represent additional side effects of larger doses of urethan.

Isopropyl carbamate is a weaker carcinogen than urethan. Twenty weeks after receiving 12 thrice-weekly intraperitoneal doses of 5 mg/dose, for a total of 60 mg, 80% of strain A/He mice had pulmonary tumors, with a mean of 1.5 tumors per animal. Isopropyl carbamate failed to demonstrate significant inhibition of DNA synthesis by 1 day although a 2-fold enhancement between 3 and 14 days was evident.

Nitrogen mustard and methylcholanthrene produced inhibition of DNA synthesis by Day 3, but no significant rebound is noted until, perhaps, at 21 days with HN2. These compounds, at the doses indicated, produce multiple pulmonary tumors in 100% of strain A/He mice (20).

Table 2

Day	Urethan (1 mg)	Urethan (0.25 mg)	Isopropyl carbamate (1 mg)	HN2[a] (0.002 mg)	MCA[a] (0.02 mg)
0	6.7[b] (5−9)		4.1 (2−8)		
1	1.7 (0−4)	5.2 (3−8)	4.7 (2−7)	4.3 (1−7)	2.2 (1−4)
3	3.0 (2−4)	3.7 (3−6)	9.2 (7−12)	1.6 (1−2)	1.5 (0−3)
5	11.0 (5−12)	5.7 (5−7)	9.0 (5−12)	4.0 (2−5)	2.7 (1−4)
8	20.2 (15−25)	3.5 (3−5)	7.7 (7−9)	3.3 (2−4)	5.7 (3−9)
14	10.2 (8−18)	7.7 (5−11)	6.0 (5−8)	3.5 (2−5)	5.2 (5−6)
21	7.5 (4−11)	3.7 (2−6	3.2 (2−5)	10.0 (9−11)	4.0 (2−6)

Thymidine index of lung cells of strain A/He mice following single exposures to 4 carcinogenic chemicals. Doses are per gm body weight; mice were killed 30 min after injection of thymidine-[3]H.

[a]HN2, methyl-bis(β-chlorethyl)-amine hydrochloride; MCA, 3-methylcholanthrene.

[b]Mean (with range indicated in parentheses), per 1000 cells.

21

EXPERIMENT 3

The availability of a wide variety of antimetabolic compounds that block the cell cycle in different phases and by acting on different synthetic pathways of nucleic acid or proteins allowed the exploration of the role of these agents on pulmonary tumor carcinogenesis in strain A mice receiving urethan.

Materials and Methods

Twelve to 15 male strain A/Jax mice, 2 months of age, were assigned at random to 6 groups as follows: (I) controls, no treatment; (II) physiologic saline, 0.1 ml; (III) actinomycin D, 0.5 μg in 0.3 ml saline; (IV) puromycin, 2.5 mg in 0.3 ml saline; (V) cytosine arabinoside, 5 mg in 0.3 ml water; and (VI) 5-fluorouracil, 2 mg in 0.4 ml of saline. All injections were subcutaneous, and in all mice of Groups II to VI, they were followed by a single intraperitoneal injection of 1 mg urethan per gm body weight. The injections of urethan were individually timed for each animal at 20 minutes after the subcutaneous injections.

Three animals from each of the 6 groups were killed at 1 hour and 24 hours after the injection of urethan, and 30 minutes following thymidine-^{3}H, as in Experiment 1. The lungs were homogenized in 0.25 M sucrose containing 5% citric acid, and the specific activity of DNA was determined by the method of Scott $et\ al.$ (16) as modified by Hinrichs $et\ al.$ (11).

The remainder of the animals, 8 to 10 per group, were maintained for 20 weeks, when they were sacrificed and the lungs fixed in Tellyesniczky's fixative. After fixation, the number of pulmonary nodules was counted for each animal.

Results

The data on the specific activity of lung DNA are given in Table 3. It is clear that urethan, at a dose of 1 mg per gm, inhibits DNA synthesis by approximately 40% at 24 hours. It is also definite that puromycin and cytosine arabinoside, at the doses and schedules used, accentuated this inhibition.

The results in regard to the lung tumor response are also indicated in Table 3. The differences between the groups are

Table 3

| Group | Treatment | Specific activity as % of control at | | Lung tumors at 20 weeks | |
		1 hr	24 hr	Lung tumors/mice	Mean no. per mouse ± S.E.
I	None	100[a]	100	2/10	0.2
II	Urethan	96	63	10/10	16.4 ± 2.7
III	Actinomycin D + urethan[b]	87	48	9/9	14.9 ± 2.0
IV	Puromycin + urethan[b]	35	30	10/10	13.2 ± 1.8
V	Cytosine arabinoside + urethan[b]	15	44	10/10	10.6 ± 2.2
VI	5-Fluorouracil + urethan[b]	109	26	8/8	21.2 ± 2.6

Effect of 5 metabolic inhibitors on pulmonary tumor induction with urethan in strain A/Jax mice.
[a] Specific activity 2300 cpm/mg DNA, 30 min after thymidine-^{3}H.
[b] 20 minutes after initial treatment.

23

not statistically significant. However, some degree of inhibition of the carcinogenic reaction may be present with cytosine arabinoside, the drug that also inhibited DNA synthesis to the greatest degree.

EXPERIMENT 4

Materials and Methods

Male mice of strains A/He, C3H, and C57BL, 2 months of age, were given urethan in single intraperitoneal doses of 1 mg per gm body weight. These strains were selected as representing animals of high, intermediate, and low susceptibility to pulmonary carcinogenesis following urethan and other carcinogenic compounds (17).

The animals were treated in a manner identical to that of Experiment 1. Three mice were killed at 1, 3, 5, 8, 14, and 21 days following urethan, and the thymidine index of alveolar cells of the lungs was determined as in Experiment 1.

Results

The results are indicated in Table 4. It shows that the initial inhibition of cell labeling occurs in each of the 3 strains. The rebound at 8 days, however, coincides with the relative susceptibility of the 3 strains, being highest for strain A/He, lower but definite for strain C3H, and not observable for strain C57BL. In all 3 strains, there is an approximate doubling of labeled cells at 21 days.

DISCUSSION

The histopathogenesis of induced primary pulmonary tumors in strain A mice is best described by Grady and Stewart (10), who used polycyclic hydrocarbons, and by Mostofi and Larsen (13), who used urethan. Both studies agree that, within 2 to 3 weeks following exposure to the carcinogen, there are focal increases of alveolar cells, particularly in subpleural and perivascular areas. These observations are corroborated by quantitative cell counts of the lungs as reported by Shimkin and Polissar (19).

The labeling of cells with tritiated thymidine following X-irradiation and urethan was reported by Foley et al. (7). There was an early depression in such labeling, which was recovered by 1 week, and this recovery was followed by a 3- to 9-fold increase in labeled cells.

The observations on thymidine-^{3}H-labeled cells appear to be in keeping with the preceding morphologic studies, adding to

24

them the early initial depression of cell labeling and thus, presumably, of DNA synthesis. It should be emphasized at this point, however, that all these studies were limited to one mouse strain, or its F_1 cross, and to one dose and schedule of carcinogen. In the case of Grady and Stewart (10), this was a single subcutaneous injection, in lard, of 0.8 mg dibenzanthracene or 1.6 mg of methylcholanthrene. Mostofi and Larsen (13) exposed the mice to an *ad libitum* access of 0.1% urethan in drinking water. Shimkin and Polissar (19) and Foley *et al.*

Table 4

	Labeled alveolar cells/1000 cells		
Days	A/He	C3H	C57BL
0	2.9	3.5	3.7
1	1.0	1.8	2.0
3	2.5	2.3	5.0
5	11.0	6.3	3.0
8	18.0	11.5	3.5
14	8.0	9.0	8.0
21	6.0	10.3	7.7

Thymidine index of alveolar cells in lungs of mice of 3 strains following single intraperitoneal dose of 1 mg urethan per gram body weight. Each point is based on 3 animals; 3000 cells were counted per mouse; all mice were killed 30 min after receiving thymidine-^{3}H.

(7) gave single intraperitoneal doses of urethan, 1 mg per gram of body weight.

Depression of DNA synthesis with chemical carginogens has been described by several investigators using different carcinogens and different animal tissues. Garcia (8) found that a single application of 0.5% 7,12-dimethylbenz(a)anthracene to the skin of newborn mice decreased the number of thymidine-^{3}H labeled cells from 0.45% to 0.1% at 24 hours. A single feeding of 15 mg DMBA to adult Sprague-Dawley rats also produced within 1 day a striking decrease in the fraction of cells in DNA synthesis in the epithelial cells of the breast and sebaceous gland (18). However, the results were similar in males and in females although females develop many more breast cancers than do males, and males develop more sebaceous gland cancers than do females. It was concluded that there was no direct relationship between eventual carcinogenic response and the initial decrease in the number of cells becoming labeled with thymidine-^{3}H.

It is of interest to recall that, in 1938, Earle and Voegtlin (5) reported that the chief effect of 3-methylcholanthrene on fibroblasts grown *in vitro* was that of severe growth retardation, at concentrations down to 2×10^{-4} mg per ml. With a series of carcinogenic agents, including urethan, polycyclic hydrocarbons, and alkylating chemicals, among the earlier tissue events is the depression of DNA synthesis as shown by thymidine-^{3}H labeling of cells. Using biochemical methods, Abell *et al.* (1) showed that the incorporation of thymidine-^{3}H into DNA, or uridine-^{3}H into total RNA, and of orotic acid-^{3}H into nuclear RNA of lung, liver, and kidney were inhibited by uracil mustard, a potent inducer of pulmonary tumors in mice. These studies were limited to 48 hours following exposure to the carcinogen.

Thus, although many carcinogens inhibit synthesis of DNA, RNA, and protein by cells, it is far from clear whether this effect is intimately involved in the process of carcinogenesis or represents yet another toxic "side effect" of the compounds. It is certainly definite that the accentuation of this initial depression of synthesis by cells of DNA, RNA, or protein by such agents as actinomycin, puromycin, or X-ray does not accentuate the carcinogenic response but the reverse. The inhibition of carcinogenesis under these circumstances is recorded for skin carcinogenesis by polycyclic hydrocarbons by Gelboin *et al.* (9), for pulmonary carcinogenesis by X-rays by Foley *et al.* (6), and by alkylating agents by Abell *et al.* (1).

It is also conceivable that damage to cellular DNA may represent an early essential step in carcinogenesis. Such damage would at first result in an inhibition of DNA synthesis, followed by an increase in the incorporation of thymidine-^{3}H into DNA due to enzymatic repair of DNA. That enzymatic repair of damaged DNA occurs in mammalian cells was shown by Rasmussen and Painter (15) in ultraviolet-damaged cells. In turn, repair of DNA would provide opportunities for pairing errors, which could lead to a carcinogenic response.

Carcinogenesis appears to be a focal reaction of tissues; that is, the eventual manifestations of neoplastic growth do not involve the whole tissue but appear as discrete and separate islands of cellular aberration. It is a relatively rare event, involving but a small proportion of the total population of cells of any tissue. Thus, crucial, specific carcinogenic reactions may be inapparent simply because they are obscured by more general reactions involving a greater proportion of the cell population. Further exploration of the synthetic processes of cells following exposure to carcinogenic agents undoubtedly will be fruitful.

It should be pointed out that such studies would be of greater value if in each instance they recognized the need for considering the dose-response relationship, the parameter of time, and the influence of the host. In other words, such investigations should be performed with several dose levels of the chemical and over a number of time periods, and should include several strains of animals of defined susceptibility to the carcinogenic reaction and some tissues from such animals that do not yield tumors as well as the tissues in which tumors are anticipated.

ACKNOWLEDGMENTS

We are indebted to the National Cancer Institute, Bethesda, Maryland, for nitrogen mustard and isopropyl carbamate. Thymidine-^{3}H was purchased from New England Nuclear Co., Boston, Massachusetts; urethan from Merck and Co., Rahway, New Jersey; and methylcholanthrene from Eastman Organic Chemicals, Rochester, New York.

ADDENDUM

Attention is directed to a paper that appeared while our report was in press: Shirley L. Kauffman. Alterations in Cell Proliferation in Mouse Lung following Urethan Exposure. I. The Nonvacuolated Alveolar Cell. Am. J. Pathol., 54: 83–93, 1969.

REFERENCES

1. Abell, C. W., Rosini, L. A., and DiPaulo, J. A. Effects of Uracil Mustard on DNA, RNA, and Protein Biosynthesis in Tissues of A/J Mice. Cancer Res., 27: 1101–1108, 1967.
2. Baserga, R. The Relationship of the Cell Cycle to Tumor Growth and Control of Cell Division: A Review. Cancer Research, 25: 581–595, 1965.
3. Baserga, R. Autoradiographic Methods. In: H. Busch (ed.), Methods in Cancer Research, Vol. 1, pp. 45–116. New York: Academic Press, Inc., 1967.
4. Baserga, R. Biochemistry of the Cell Cycle: A Review. Cell and Tissue Kinetics, 1: 167–191, 1968.
5. Earle, W. R., and Voegtlin, C. The Mode of Action of Methylcholanthrene on Cultures of Normal Tissues. Am. J. Cancer, 34: 373–390, 1938.
6. Foley, W. A., and Cole, L. J. Inhibition of Urethane Lung Tumor Induction in Mice by Total-Body X-Radiation. Cancer Res., 23: 1176–1180, 1963.
7. Foley, W. A., Cole, L. J., Ingram, B. J., and Crocker, T. T. X-ray Inhibition of Urethan-stimulated Proliferation of Lung Cells of the Mouse as Estimated by Incorporation of Tritiated Thymidine. Nature, 199: 1267–68, 1963.
8. Garcia, H. Intake of Tritiated Thymidine by Epidermal Cells of

Newborn Mice Treated with 7,12-Dimethylbenz(a)anthracene. Exptl. Cell Res., 27: 182–185, 1962.

9. Gelboin, H. V., Klein, M., and Bates, R. R. Inhibition of Mouse Skin Tumorigenesis by Actinomycin D. Proc. Natl. Acad. Sci. U. S., 53: 1353–1360, 1965.

10. Grady, H. G., and Stewart, H. L. Histogenesis of Induced Pulmonary Tumors in Strain A Mice. Am. J. Pathol., 16: 417–432, 1940.

11. Hinrichs, H. R., Petersen, R. O., and Baserga, R. Incorporation of Thymidine Into DNA of Mouse Organs. Arch. Pathol., 70: 245–253, 1964.

12. Mirvish, S. S. The Carcinogenic Action and Metabolism of Urethane and N-nydroxyurethan. Advan. Cancer Res., in press.

13. Mostofi, F. K., and Larsen, C. D. The Histopathogenesis of Pulmonary Tumors Induced in Strain A Mice by Urethane. J. Natl. Cancer Inst., 11: 1187–1222, 1951.

14. Neyman, J., and Scott, E. L. Statistical Aspects of the Problem of Carcinogenesis. Proc. Fifth Berkeley Symposium on Mathematical Statistics and Probability, Vol. 4, pp. 745–776. Berkeley: Univ. Calif. Press, 1967.

15. Rasmussen, R. E., and Painter, R. B. Evidence for Repair of Ultraviolet Damaged Deoxyribonucleic Acid in Cultured Mammalian Cells. Nature, 203: 1360–1362, 1964.

16. Scott, J. F., Franccastoro, A. P., and Taft, E. B. Studies in Histochemistry ± Determination of Nucleic Acids in Microgram Amounts of Tissue. J. Histochem. Cytochem., 4: 1–10, 1956.

17. Shimkin, M. B. Pulmonary Tumors in Experimental Animals. Advan. Cancer Res., 3: 223–267, 1955.

18. Shimkin, M. B., Gruenstein, M., Thatcher, D. and Baserga, R. Tritiated Thymidine Labeling of Cells in Rats Following Exposure to 7,12-Dimethylbenz(a)anthracene. Cancer Res., 27: 1494–1495, 1967.

19. Shimkin, M. B., and Polissar, M. J. Some Quantitative Observations on the Induction and Growth of Primary Pulmonary Tumors in Strain A Mice Receiving Urethane. J. Natl. Cancer Inst., 16: 75–97, 1955.

20. Shimkin, M. B., Weisburger, J. H., Weisburger, E. K., Gubareff, N., and Suntzeff, V. Bioassay of 29 Alkylating Chemicals by the Pulmonary-Tumor Response in Strain A Mice. J. Natl. Cancer Inst., 26: 915–935, 1966.

21. Shimkin, M. B., Wieder, R., Marzi, D., Gubareff, N., and Suntzeff, V. Lung Tumors in Mice Receiving Different Schedules of Urethane. Proc. Fifth Berkeley Symposium on Mathematical Statistics and Probability, pp. 707–719. Berkeley: Univ. Calif. Press, 1967.

QUANTITATIVE STUDIES ON THE MALIGNANT TRANSFORMATION OF MOUSE PROSTATE CELLS BY CARCINOGENIC HYDROCARBONS *IN VITRO*

by

T. T. CHEN and Charles HEIDELBERGER

In this laboratory we have long been concerned with the cellular and molecular mechanisms whereby polycyclic aromatic hydrocarbons initiate the process of carcinogenesis (Heidelberger, 1964; Heidelberger and Giovanella, 1966). This research has largely involved measurements of the *in vivo* binding of hydrocarbons of differing carcinogenic activities to the proteins (Abell and Heidelberger, 1962) and nucleic acids (Goshman and Heidelberger, 1967) of mouse skin, following topical application of the labelled compounds. The limitation to experiments imposed by working with whole animals has led us to search for a system that would make possible quantitative studies of hydrocarbon carcinogenesis *in vitro*. We followed the lead provided by Lasnitzki (1963), who treated organ cultures of mouse ventral prostate with methylcholanthrene (MCA) and obtained histological changes suggestive of neoplasia. With modification of her techniques we were able to obtain profound morphological changes that resembled those of carcinogenesis by treating C3H mouse ventral prostates in organ culture with various hydrocarbons (Röller and Heidelberger, 1967). However, in order to determine whether carcinogenesis *in vitro* had actually occurred, we implanted 872 of such morphologically altered pieces into as many mice under a variety of conditions without obtaining any tumors. But when the prostate pieces that had been treated with carcinogenic hydrocarbons in organ culture were dispersed with pronase and grown in cell culture, a number of permanent cell lines were obtained that exhibited all the criteria of malignancy, including the ability to produce tumors on inoculation into C3H mice (Heidelberger and Iype, 1967, 1968. Thus carcinogenesis *in vitro* had been accomplished, but we lacked long-term cell lines from untreated organ cultures that could have proved that the transformations we observed were actually produced by the carcinogens and not by the process of spontaneous malignant transformation that is quite ubiquitous in long-term cultures of mouse cells (*cf.* Sanford, 1968). In subsequent work, however, we were successful in obtaining cell lines derived from organ cultures of untreated mouse prostates, which underwent spontaneous malignant transformation rarely and only after more than 250 days in culture (Chen and Heidelberger, 1968, 1969a, 1969b). These cell lines, although aneuploid, were highly " contact inhibited " before the time of spontaneous malignant transformation, i.e. they grew as a monolayer and after reaching a saturation density did not pile up and grow further (Chen and Heidelberger, 1969a) under standard conditions of nutrition. Moreover, they were sensitive to the toxicity of carcinogenic hydrocarbons, and grew maximally only in media enriched with 10% fetal calf serum. When methylcholanthrene at 0.5 and 1.0 μg/ml was added to these cells for six days and the culture was continued in carcinogen-free medium, morphologically distinct colonies of randomly oriented piled-up cells that stained very deeply with Giemsa were formed (Chen and Heidelberger, 1968, 1969b). When the cells were isolated from such colonies they were found, in contrast to the control cells, to grow in a multilayer fashion with no saturation density under the same conditions; they were resistant to the toxicity of carcinogenic hydrocarbons; and they grew at optimal rates in media containing 1.0% fetal calf serum (Chen and Heidelberger, 1969b). More important, however, was the fact that a 100% incidence of fibrosarcomas resulted when as few as 1,000 cells were inoculated subcutaneously into unconditioned C3H mice, whereas the control cells taken after the same period in culture produced no tumors when more than 10^6 cells were inoculated into previously X-irradiated mice (Chen and Heidelberger, 1969b).

Thus, carcinogenesis *in vitro* with hydrocarbons was accomplished by us under conditions and at times where no spontaneous malignant transformation occurred. The distinctive appearance of the piled-up transformed colonies has made it possible for us to quantitate the system, and this forms the substance of the present report. Throughout this paper the word " transformation " is used purely as an operational term, with no implications as to mechanism.

During the course of our research a number of reports have appeared that describe varying degrees of success in obtaining chemical carcinogenesis *in vitro*. These include the papers of Berwald and Sachs (1965), Borenfreund et al. (1966), Sanders and Burford (1967), DiPaolo and Donovan (1967), and Kuroki and Sato (1968). Borek and Sachs (1966a) have also been able to achieve morphological transformation by X-irradiation, but these cells did not give rise to progressively growing tumors on inoculation into hamsters. A number of other papers dealing with various aspects of chemical carcinogenesis *in vitro* have been published from Sachs' laboratory, and some will be specifically referred to later (Borek and Sachs, 1966b; Huberman and Sachs, 1966). In most of the studies referred to above, cells derived from embryonic mouse or hamster fibroblasts were used, whereas in our research we have employed a cell line derived from an adult differentiated tissue.

MATERIAL AND METHODS

Cell culture

All cell cultures were incubated at 37° C in humidified incubators with a gas phase of air: carbon dioxide 95:5. Falcon plastic dishes, 35 mm with 2 ml, or 65 mm with 5 ml of media, were used throughout. The medium was Eagle's BME (Eagle, 1959) plus 10% fetal calf serum, which were obtained from the Grand Island Biological Laboratories (Grand Island, N.Y., USA). The Bl prostate cells, obtained from organ cultures of adult C3H mouse ventral prostates and used in these experiments (Chen and Heidelberger, 1969a) had been transferred for 16 to 28 subcultures (120-180 days) and were aneuploid. Most of them were taken from the frozen state at the time of the experiments. Under the standard conditions for the quantitative experiments, 1,000 Bl cells were plated in 35 mm plastic dishes on a feeder layer

30

of C3H mouse embryonic fibroblasts that had been irradiated with 5,000 R and prepared according to the method of Puck and Marcus (1955). One day after plating, hydrocarbon-containing medium with a final concentration of 0.5% dimethyl sulfoxide (DMSO) is added to the culture and incubated for 6 days, during which time there are two medium changes. The hydrocarbons are then washed out of the cultures and carcinogen-free medium is added. Two days later some of the dishes are fixed with methanol and stained with Giemsa, and the colonies are counted in order to determine the overall plating efficiency. Control cultures are similarly treated with 0.5% DMSO. Other replicate dishes are kept an additional 2-3 weeks, with medium changes every 2-3 days, and are then fixed, stained, and scored for piled-up (transformed) colonies.

Hydrocarbons used

The carcinogenic hydrocarbons used in these experiments included: 3,4-benzpyrene (BP), 3-methylcholanthrene (MCA), 9,10-dimethyl-1,2-benzanthracene (DMBA), 1,2,5,6-dibenzanthracene (1,2,5,6-DBA), and 4-fluoro-10-methyl-1,2-benzanthracene (4-F-10-Me-BA). The non-carcinogenic hydrocarbons used were: 1,2,3,4-dibenzanthracene (1,2,3,4-DBA), 3-fluoro-10-methyl-1,2-benzanthracene (3-F-10-Me-BA), and pyrene. All compounds were dissolved in DMSO as a stock solution, kept shielded from the light, and then the appropriate amount of the stock solution was added to the protein-containing medium (the protein solubilizes the compounds) to give a final DMSO concentration of 0.5%, which does not affect the growth of these cells. These hydrocarbons were obtained from various commercial sources, and 3-F-10-Me-BA and 4-F-10-Me-BA were generously donated by Dr. J. A. Miller of this laboratory.

Tumorigenicity tests

Piled-up colonies were located in the dishes by phase contrast microscopy, and individually isolated by the ring isolation technique (Puck *et al.*, 1956) (a small glass tube, 3 mm inside diameter, that is treated on its lower surface with silicone stopcock grease is carefully placed over the colony to isolate it from its surroundings, 0.1 ml of 0.05% trypsin is added, and after 10 min at 37° C the cells are detached from the dish with gentle pipetting and transferred out of the tube).

Viable cells remaining in a monolayer were isolated from the carcinogen-treated dishes by the same technique. The various cells were counted in a hemocytometer or a Coulter counter, Model B, and suspended in 0.1 ml of medium, which was then injected directly into the brains of C3H mice.

Male C3H mice (A. R. Schmidt Co., Madison, Wis., USA), weighing approximately 25 g, were used for all of the injections. Approximately 0.25 ml of a 5 mg/ml solution of Nembutal sodium (Abbott Laboratories), diluted in physiological saline, was injected intraperitoneally to anesthetize the animals. The mice were secured on a table and their heads cleaned with 80% alcohol. A small incision (10 mm) was made at the base of the skull to expose the brain. At about 1 mm to the left of the median, the skull was penetrated with a Bard Parker no. 11 blade. The blade was then withdrawn and the cell suspension was injected through this opening, using a tuberculin syringe with a 26 gauge needle, at a 45° angle and at a depth of 5-7 mm. Neosporin powder (Burroughs Wellcome & Co.) was applied to the entire open area and two or three 9 mm stainless steel wound clips were used to close the incision. The mortality was very low with this procedure. When tumors were obtained, they protruded through the opening in the skull. Mice were held for 180 days before being scored as negative for palpable tumors.

RESULTS

The gross appearances of fixed and stained dishes containing the monolayer of control cells and piled-up transformed colonies are shown in Figure 1.

In order to establish the optimal conditions for the quantitative assay of the morphological transformation of mouse prostate cells, a number of preliminary experiments were carried out. One of these, summarized in Table I, shows that the highest transformation percentage occurred at the lowest cell density of 5×10^2 cells/ml in 2 ml of medium in a 35 mm dish. No difference was found between the frequencies of transformation in 35 or 65 mm dishes, and the former were used subsequently for reasons of convenience and economy. It was shown in other experiments that the overall plating efficiency for 1,000 cells was somewhat higher (5.0%) when a feeder layer was used than when it was not (3.6%). Therefore, the standard assay system adopted involved plating

31

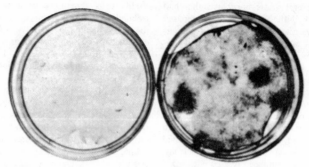

FIGURE 1

Photographs of fixed and Giemsa-stained dishes of control, DMSO-treated prostate cells (left) and methylcholanthrene-treated cultures (right). These were fixed and stained after the following treatment: 1 day after plating the dishes were treated for 6 days with 0.5% DMSO or 1 μg/ml of MCA, after which they were cultured 2 additional weeks in carcinogen-free medium and then fixed and stained. Individual transformed colonies are seen in the right-hand dish, and the monolayer of lightly-stained cells in the left-hand dish is only faintly seen.

TABLE I

THE EFFECT OF PLATING DIFFERENT DENSITIES OF PROSTATE CELLS
(WITHOUT FEEDER LAYER) ON TRANSFORMATION

Density cells/ml	Treatment	No. transformed colonies/ No. dishes	% Transformation based on number of cells plated
5×10^4	DMSO	0/4	0
5×10^4	MCA, 1 μg/ml	28/4	0.007
5×10^3	DMSO	0/4	0
5×10^3	MCA, 1 μg/ml	9/4	0.022
5×10^2	DMSO	0/4	0
5×10^2	MCA, 1 μg/ml	5/4	0.13

The prostate cells were taken at the 17th subculture (126 days), and the experiment was carried out in 2 ml of medium in 35 mm dishes. The treatment was started 1 day after plating, and continued for 6 days. The piled-up transformed colonies were scored 2 weeks later.

1,000 Bl prostate cells in 2 ml of medium in 35 mm dishes on a feeder layer of mouse embryonic cells. Table I also shows that morphologically transformed, piled-up colonies that are deeply stained with Giemsa were consistently produced by methylcholanthrene (MCA) whereas none were observed in the control cultures (including all subsequent experiments).

The time sequence adopted for the quantitative experiments is described under Material and Methods. The essence of the procedure involves scoring for total colonies (overall plating effi-ciency) 8 days after plating, and for transformed colonies in other dishes 2-3 weeks later when these colonies had piled up on top of a monolayer of untransformed cells. The scoring was aided by fixing and staining the dishes. Figure 2 shows the microscopic appearance of a deeply-stained piled-up colony in the dish shown in Figure 1, together with the adjacent monolayer area. Figure 3 shows a monolayer, untransformed area of the same MCA-treated dish. Thus, it is evident that in this system, scoring for transformed colonies is quite unambiguous.

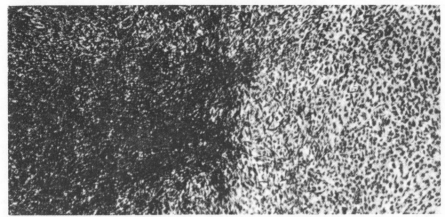

FIGURE 2

Photomicrograph (45×) of the edge of one of the piled-up transformed colonies in the right-hand dish of Figure 1. The deeply-stained piled-up array of cells in the transformed colony is evident, and contrasts witht he strict monolayer orientation of the cells outside the colony.

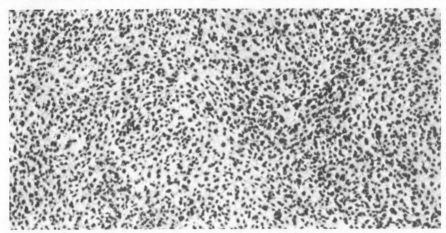

FIGURE 3

Photomicrograph (45×) of a monolayer area in the MCA-treated dish of Figure 1. The appearance of untreated or DMSO control dishes is identical. It is such an area that was isolated (located by phase-contrast) and used for the experiment described in Table II.

Tumor production by the cells isolated from piled-up colonies and monolayer areas in the same dishes

We have thus far described the production with MCA of piled-up colonies that have undergone morphological transformation. We have pre-

viously reported (Chen and Heidelberger, 1969b) that cells from mass cultures of MCA-treated prostate cells that contained piled-up colonies gave fibrosarcomas on inoculation into isologous mice. In order to determine whether in the presently described system morphological trans-

33

TABLE II

INOCULATION OF INDIVIDUAL PILED-UP COLONIES AND MONOLAYER AREAS
INTO THE BRAINS OF C3H MICE

Dish No.	Type of area isolated	No. cells inoculated/ mouse	No. mice	Duration of observation days	Times of tumor appearance days	No. tumors
1	Monolayer	1,000	4	150	—	0
1	Piled-up	1,000	3	90	30-90	3
1	Piled-up	100	3	150	30-150	2
1	Piled-up	10	3	150	36	1
2	Monolayer	1,000	3	60	—	0
2	Piled-up Colony 1	500	3	60	30-60	3
2	Piled-up Colony 2	500	3	60	30	1
2	Piled-up Colony 3	500	3	60	30	1
2	Piled-up Colony 4	500	3	60	30	1
2	Piled-up Colony 5	500	3	60	30-60	2
2	Piled-up Colony 6	500	3	60	30-60	2

MCA at 1 μg/ml was added to each dish. Each experiment represents one 35 mm dish. For description, see text.

formation can be equated with malignant transformation it was necessary to see whether individual colonies could produce tumors in mice. Accordingly, in two dishes, individual piled-up colonies were located by phase-contrast microscopy and ring isolated. Monolayer areas from the same MCA-treated dishes were similarly isolated. All of these isolates were passaged once in culture in order to obtain enough cells to inject, and the cells derived from the piled-up colonies and the monolayer areas grew equally well. The cells derived from these subcultures were then injected directly into the brains of C3H mice, with the results shown in Table II. This experiment shows clearly that as few as 10 cells isolated from the morphologically transformed colonies produced tumors, that all nine transformed colonies tested in this experiment gave rise to tumors, and that 1,000 cells derived from the monolayer areas of the carcinogen-treated dishes (and which grew well in the subculture) induced no tumors. These tumors, and others induced in this system, were histologically diagnosed as malignant fibrosarcomas, tumors that are progressively growing and kill the mice, are readily transplanted, and under some circumstances can metastasize. Such experiments have been repeated several times and are reproducible. Thus, it has been established that in this system morphological transformation is equated with malignant transformation, and that regardless of the exact mechanism, carcinogenesis in vitro has really been achieved. Furthermore, it is likely from these data that all piled-up colonies contain malignant cells, and that the monolayer areas of viable cells in control or treated dishes do not contain malignant cells. Therefore, the quantitation of malignant transformation by counting the number of piled-up colonies in fixed and stained dishes is completely justified.

Effects of various concentrations of hydrocarbons on malignant transformation

In order to determine whether the ability of a series of hydrocarbons to produce in vitro malignant transformation parallels carcinogenic activity, a dose-response experiment was carried out with eight hydrocarbons. The results are plotted in Figures 4-6 and tabulated in Table III. With those compounds that produced transformed colonies, the logarithm of the number of transformed colonies per 7,000 cells plated (seven dishes) is plotted against the logarithm of the concentration of the hydrocarbon maintained in the medium for 6 days. For each compound, the relative plating efficiency, which is a measure of toxicity, is also plotted as determined with five dishes for each point. The time sequence of the experiment is described in Material and Methods. It is evident that there is an excellent correlation between the carcinogenic activity (more precisely the initiating activity in the two-stage system on mouse skin) of the compounds and their ability to produce in vitro malignant transformation in this system. The powerful carcinogens 9,10-dimethyl-1,2-benzanthracene (DMBA) and 4-fluoro-10-methyl-1,2-benzanthracene (4-F-10-Me-BA) (Fig. 4), and 3,4-benzpyrene (BP) and 3-methylcholanthrene (MCA) (Fig. 5) produced maximum transformation frequencies of 26, 35, 28, and 16/7,000 cells, respectively. The moderately active initiator, 1,2,5,6-dibenzanthracene (1,2,5,6-DBA) (Fig. 6) produced four transformed colonies/seven dishes, and the noncarcinogenic 1,2,3,4-dibenzanthracene (1,2,3,4-DBA), 3-fluoro-10-methyl-1,2-benzanthracene (3-F-10-Me-BA) and pyrene (Table III) did not give rise to *any* transformed colonies. Consequently, this system may eventually find some use as an alternative screening method for determining carcinogenic activity in the hydrocarbon series (other classes of chemical carcinogens have not yet been tested in this system). In the case of all the hydrocarbons that produced transformations, there was an optimal concentration above which the transformation frequency diminished. The reason for this decrease is not yet understood.

The toxicity exerted by the various compounds, expressed as plating efficiency relative to the DMSO controls, is also plotted in Figures 4-6 and given in Table III. It is evident that there is no simple relationship between the transforming activity of the various compounds and the toxicity they exert. As shown in Table III, the noncarcinogenic hydrocarbons are toxic to these

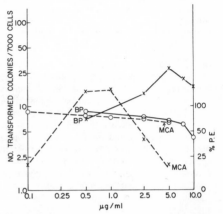

FIGURE 5

The transformation frequencies and toxicities produced by different concentrations of BP and MCA added to the media for 6 days. For further information, see the legend to Figure 4.

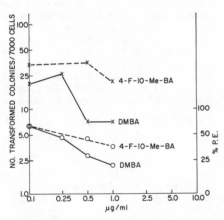

FIGURE 4

The transformation frequencies and toxicities produced by different concentrations of DMBA and 4-F-10-Me-BA added to the media for 6 days. For abbreviations, see text. This is a double-logarithmic plot. The X points correspond to the transformation frequencies, and the 0 points correspond to the plating efficiencies relative to the controls (determined in four dishes for each point). The overall plating efficiency of the DMSO controls was 5.3%. The Bl cells used in this experiment were taken at the 16th subculture.

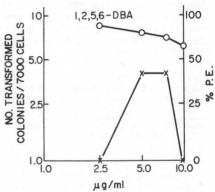

FIGURE 6

The transformation frequencies and toxicities produced by different concentrations of 1,2,5,6-DBA added to the media for 6 days. For further information, see the legend to Figure 4.

35

TABLE III

THE INACTIVITY OF NON-CARCINOGENIC HYDROCARBONS IN *IN VITRO* TRANSFORMATION
For conditions, see text.

Compound	Concentration μg/ml	Plating efficiency %	No. transformed colonies / No. dishes
DMSO control	0.5%	5.3	0/10
1,2,3,4-Dibenzanthracene	1.0	4.2 (79%)	0/7
1,2,3,4-Dibenzanthracene	5.0	2.8 (53%)	0/7
3-Fluoro-10-methyl-1,2-benzanthracene	1.0	4.3	0/7
3-Fluoro-10-methyl-1,2-benzanthracene	5.0	3.6 (68%)	0/7
3-Fluoro-10-methyl-1,2-benzanthracene	10.0	3.0 (57%)	0/7
Pyrene	1.0	4.6 (87%)	0/8

cells, but do not transform them. Although there is some parallelism between toxicity and transformation with DMBA and 4-F-10-Me-BA (Fig. 4), there is none in the case of BP and MCA (Fig. 5) and 1,2,5,6-DBA (Fig. 6). Huberman and Sachs (1966) also reached the conclusion that the toxicity exerted by and the transformation produced by BP probably represent different processes. It is clear that toxicity alone cannot explain the decreased transformation frequencies produced by the hydrocarbons at higher concentrations in our experiments.

Malignant transformation after treatment for different times with MCA

The purpose of these experiments was to determine whether malignant transformation would occur if the cells were treated with the hydrocarbons for less than 6 days. As shown in Table IV, higher concentrations of MCA than the optimal level for 6-day treatment were added one day after plating on a feeder layer, and were washed out after 1 and 2 days and replaced with carcinogen-free medium. The highest frequency of transformation occurred with 1 day's treatment with MCA at 10 μg/ml, and the transformation frequency decreased at higher concentrations. Further experiments were carried out as shown in Table V. At the lowest level of MCA the transformation frequency was highest after treatment for 6-8 days. However, with increasingly higher concentrations the optimal time of treatment became shorter. Thus, it is possible to obtain relatively high transformation frequencies by treatment with hydrocarbon for only 1 day. This may make it possible to calculate true transformation efficiencies, since the number of cells present during such an interval can be determined. For example, in the experiment in Table IV where the cells were treated with MCA for 1 day at 10 μg/ml 1 day after plating, the true transformation frequency was: $\dfrac{11 \times 100}{0.038 \times 3000} = 9.6\%$. This calculation involves the assumption that the

TABLE IV

TRANSFORMATION FREQUENCIES AND PLATING EFFICIENCIES PRODUCED IN CONTROL
(B1, TAKEN AT THE 16th SUBCULTURE) PROSTATE CELLS BY TREATMENT WITH MCA FOR 1 AND 2 DAYS
A feeder layer was used and the MCA was added 1 day after plating.

Treatment	Plating efficiency [1] %		No. Transformed colonies / No. dishes	
	1 day	2 days	1 day	2 days
DMSO	5.2	5.1	0/3	0/3
MCA, 5 μg/ml	4.1	3.5	5/3	8/3
MCA, 10 μg/ml	3.8	3.2	11/3	4/3
MCA, 15 μg/ml	3.4	3.1	6/3	1/3
MCA, 20 μg/ml	3.4	2.9	3/3	1/3

[1] Determined in 3 dishes for each value.

TABLE V

EFFECT OF DIFFERENT DURATION OF TREATMENT WITH MCA ON THE
TRANSFORMATION FREQUENCY OF B1 PROSTATE CELLS TAKEN AT THE 18th SUBCULTURE
The MCA was added 1 day after plating.

Treatment	No. transformed colonies/7 dishes				
Duration of treatment (days):	1	2	3	6	8
DMSO	—[1]	—	—	—	0
MCA, 1 μg/ml	11	12	15	30	30
MCA, 5 μg/ml	19	19	12	6	—
MCA, 10 μg/ml	22	22	9	—	—
MCA, 15 μg/ml	23	21	10	—	—
MCA, 20 μg/ml	19	13	4	—	—

[1] —. not done.

hydrocarbon exerted its effect during the time it was added, although it is recognized that because of binding to cell constituents, this is not a true pulse.

The effect of 1-day treatment with MCA at different times after plating

In this experiment, 1,000 control cells were plated on a feeder layer, and 10 μg/ml of MCA was added on the 1st, 2nd, 3rd, 6th and 8th days after plating. The free hydrocarbon was washed out after one day, and the scoring of transformed colonies was as before. Table VI shows that the transformation frequency was highest when the carcinogen was added on the first day after plating, and diminished when the MCA was added later, so that no transformation was

obtained when the hydrocarbon was added on the 8th day.

Borek and Sachs (1967) demonstrated that with cells morphologically transformed by X-irradiation cell division was necessary to " fix " the transformed state. It appears from the experiment shown in Table VI that the same requirement for cell division to fix the transformation holds in our system, since no transformed colonies were obtained when the MCA was added on the 8th day after plating at which time the cells were in a confluent monolayer. Further investigation of this point is currently under way in our laboratory.

The effect of heat treatment on the control and transformed cells

We have recently become interested in the selective lethal effects of heat on cancer cells from the biological, biochemical, and clinical points of view (Cavaliere *et al.*, 1967; Giovanella and Heidelberger, 1968). Therefore, it was of interest to test the lethal effects of heat on our control and transformed cells. Three days after plating, the control cells and a line of cells recently transformed from them were incubated at 43° C for various periods of time, and their plating efficiencies relative to 37° C were plotted against time, as shown in Figure 7. It is clear that the viability of the control cells was not significantly affected by this heat treatment, which did exert a considerable killing effect on the transformed cells. A comparison of the treatment of the control and transformed cells for 90 min at various temperatures is given in Figure 8, and the greatest difference in killing of the two cell types was found

TABLE VI

TRANSFORMATION FREQUENCIES PRODUCED BY
1-DAY TREATMENT WITH MCA (10 μg/ml)
ADDED AT DIFFERENT TIMES AFTER PLATING
B1 prostate cells were used at the 19th subculture.

Time of addition of hydro-carbon, days after plating	No. transformed colonies No. dishes	
	DMSO	MCA
1st	0/10	40/10
2nd	0/10	27/10
3rd	0/10	8/8
6th	0/10	3/10
8th	0/10	0/10

The scoring was done two weeks after the day of treatment with MCA.

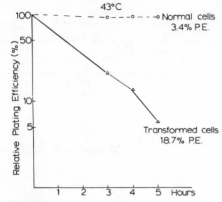

FIGURE 7

The effect of heat treatment at 43° C on the relative plating efficiencies of control and transformed cells. For conditions, see the text and the legend to Table VII. The overall plating efficiencies of the cells are given in the graph.

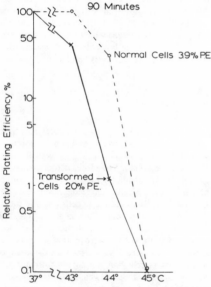

FIGURE 8

The effect of heating for 90 min at various temperatures on the relative plating efficiencies of control and transformed cells. For conditions, see text and the legend to Table VII. The overall plating efficiencies of the cells are given on the graph.

at 44° C. Thus, it appears that the acquisition of sensitivity to the lethal effects of heat is an early property of the *in vitro* transformation of these cells, or else that only heat-sensitive cells were transformed.

This question was resolved by the experiment shown in Table VII. When control cells were pre-heated at 42.5° C for 4 hours prior to the transformation experiment, they were transformed by MCA with the same efficiency as the non-heated cells. Therefore, the acquisition of sensitivity to the lethal effects of heat is an early property of transformation in this system, and is in accord with the heat sensitivity of cancer cells previously determined (Cavaliere *et al.*, 1967). Whether this is a general phenomenon remains to be seen, because Ossovski and Sachs (1967) have found that cells transformed by a strain of polyoma virus are more stable to heat than the untransformed cells. However, Sachs (personal communication) has also found that chemically and X-ray-transformed hamster cells show increased sensitivity to the lethal effects of heat.

TABLE VII

THE EFFECT OF HEAT TREATMENT OF CONTROL PROSTATE CELLS PRIOR TO THE TRANSFORMATION EXPERIMENT

Conditions	Plating efficiency %	No. transformed cells/5,000 cells plated
Non-heated DMSO	5.5	0
Non-heated MCA, 1 μg/ml	3.8	36
Heated [1] DMSO	5.3	0
Heated [1] MCA, 1 μg/ml	3.6	33

[1] The cells were heated 4 days after plating at 42.5° C for 4 hours. They were then kept overnight at 37° C and plated for the transformation experiment. The B1 prostate cells were taken at the 17th subculture and treated with DMSO or MCA. After isolation of the piled-up colonies, the MCA-treated cells were subcultured once and taken for this experiment at the second subculture. Similarly, the DMSO cells were taken at the subculture after DMSO treatment. Thus, both cell sublines were cultured for the same length of time.

DISCUSSION

Our previous studies on the malignant transformation of C3H mouse ventral prostate cells by carcinogenic hydrocarbons *in vitro* (for references, see page 178) have now been extended to the point where a system has been developed that is reproducible and quantitative under conditions and at times where spontaneous malignant transformation does not occur. Aneuploid cell lines derived from adult C3H mouse ventral prostate are plated at a density of 1,000 cells in 35 mm plastic dishes on a feeder layer of C3H mouse embryo fibroblasts and treated with 0.5% dimethyl sulfoxide or solutions of hydrocarbons in 0.5% DMSO. Eight days after plating some of the dishes are fixed and stained, and the total colonies are counted to give the overall plating efficiency. The other dishes are kept for an additional 2-3 weeks and then are fixed and stained. The control cells grow to a confluent monolayer and reach a saturation density. The cultures treated with carcinogenic hydrocarbons form piled-up multilayered colonies that stain darkly with Giemsa and can readily be scored to give transformation frequency (Fig. 1). It has been shown previously (Chen and Heidelberger, 1969b) that the control cells, at the time they are used for the transformation experiments, do not give rise to tumors when more than 10^6 cells are injected subcutaneously into adult irradiated C3H mice, whereas the transformed cells give a 100% incidence of malignant fibrosarcomas when as few as 1,000 cells are inoculated subcutaneously into adult unconditioned C3H mice. In order to justify the conclusion that the piled-up colonies that we score as transformed are really malignant, experiments have been done that show that every such colony in a dish is capable of giving tumors when injected into the brains of C3H mice, whereas the viable cells obtained from the monolayer areas of the same carcinogen-treated dishes do not give tumors.

Very recently, Aaronson and Todaro (1968) have found a similar parallelism between the malignancy of mouse cells in culture and their ability to grow in crowded cultures, a property exhibited as piled-up colonies.

Among all the other reports on chemical carcinogenesis in vitro (see pages 177-178) only those of Berwald and Sachs (1965) and subsequent papers from that laboratory report quantitative studies comparable to our present ones. However, they have not published any experiments to determine whether the individual colonies that they score are actually malignant. The only tumors that they report (Berwald and Sachs, 1965) were derived from mass cultures and not individual colonies.

It is also of interest that Berwald and Sachs (1965) judged their transformed colonies at the time we score plating efficiencies and before they have the opportunity to pile up, thus requiring eyes attuned to morphological subtleties. In our system, the scoring for transformation is delayed until the transformed colonies have piled up on the underlying monolayer; thus, scoring is quite unambiguous. Furthermore, we do not believe that it is justifiable to calculate transformation efficiencies by dividing the transformation frequency by the plating efficiency as Berwald and Sachs (1965) and Huberman and Sachs (1966) have done. The reason is that the carcinogen is present for one week in the culture, and if the transformation took place at a distinct time during that week, we do not know how many cells were present in the culture at that particular time, since they increase in number throughout the culture period and the colony count only scores for the number of cells originally plated.

There is an excellent quantitative correlation between the carcinogenic (or initiating) activity of eight hydrocarbons and the frequency with which they produce malignant transformation in this system. Berwald and Sachs (1965) also found such a correlation. Although, in most of our experiments, the carcinogen was added to the cultures for 6 days, it has also been possible to produce transformation by a 1-day treatment with the hydrocarbons.

The question may be asked whether our control untransformed cells are really normal. Actually, they are aneuploid (Chen and Heidelberger, 1969a), so that they cannot be considered to be completely normal. Yet, under the conditions of our experiments, they reach a saturation density and do not multiply further once a monolayer is formed. The control cells are also susceptible to the toxicity of carcinogenic hydrocarbons, as found by Borek and Sachs (1966b) for their embryonic hamster fibroblasts, and they do not give tumors even in irradiated mice. Furthermore, they require 10% serum for optimal growth, and Temin (1967) has found that there is a greater requirement for a serum factor (partially purified by Holley and Kiernan, 1968) by normal chick fibroblasts than there is for such cells transformed by the Rous sarcoma virus. Therefore, our control cells have some of the properties of normal cells. Whether aneuploidy is required for successful malignant transformation by chemical carcinogens is not yet known. Again, it should be emphasized that we have used the word "transformation" without any implications concerning mechanism.

The finding that the acquisition of sensitivity to the lethal effects of heat is an early consequence of malignant transformation is of considerable interest, but its generality as a fundamental property of malignant cells requires further investigation.

With this system it should now be possible to determine which of the following cellular mechanisms obtain with hydrocarbon carcinogenesis: 1) the carcinogen transforms normal cells into cancer cells; 2) the carcinogen selects for pre-existing cancer cells, as proposed by Prehn (1964); 3) the carcinogen activates a latent oncogenic virus. The question of the activation of a latent oncogenic virus is a complicated one. Considerable negative evidence had been accumulated (Heidelberger and Iype, 1967) in earlier work with different cell lines. We have not as yet examined this system for the presence or activation of a latent oncogenic virus. It is hoped that further research will clarify these matters and establish the cellular mechanism of hydrocarbon carcinogenesis before the molecular mechanisms can be effectively approached.

ACKNOWLEDGEMENTS

This work was supported in part by grants CA-7175 and CRTY-5002 from the National Cancer Institute, National Institutes of Health, US Public Health Service. We are grateful to Mrs. Lois Griesbach and Mr. Bernard Biales for skilled technical assistance.

C.H. is an American Cancer Society Professor of Oncology.

REFERENCES

AARONSON, S. A., and TODARO, G. J., Basis for the acquisition of malignant potential by mouse cells cultivated in vitro. Science, 162, 1024-1026 (1968).

ABELL, C. W., and HEIDELBERGER, C., The interaction of carcinogenic hydrocarbons with tissues. VIII. Binding of tritium-labeled hydrocarbons to the soluble proteins of mouse skin. Cancer Res., 22, 931-946 (1962).

BERWALD, Y., and SACHS, L., In vitro transformation of normal cells into tumor cells by carcinogenic hydrocarbons. J. nat. Cancer Inst., 35, 641-661 (1965).

BOREK, C., and SACHS, L., *In vitro* cell transformation by X-irradiation. *Nature (Lond.)*, **210**, 276-278 (1966a).

BOREK, C., and SACHS, L., The difference in contact inhibition of cell replication between normal cells and cells transformed by different carcinogens. *Proc. nat. Acad. Sci. (Wash.)*, **56**, 1705-1711 (1966b).

BOREK, C., and SACHS, L., Cell susceptibility to transformation by X-irradiation and fixation of the transformed state. *Proc. nat. Acad. Sci. (Wash.)*, **57**, 1522-1527 (1967).

BORENFREUND, E., KRIM, M., SANDERS, F. K., STERNBERG, S. S., and BENDICH, A., Malignant conversion of cells *in vitro* by carcinogens and viruses. *Proc. nat. Acad. Sci. (Wash.)*, **56**, 672-679 (1966).

CAVALIERE, R., CIOCATTO, E. C., GIOVANELLA, B. C., HEIDELBERGER, C., JOHNSON, R. O., MARGOTTINI, M., MONDIVI, B., MORICCA, G., and ROSSI-FANELLI, A., Selective heat sensitivity of cancer cells. Biochemical and clinical studies. *Cancer*, **20**, 1351-1381 (1967).

CHEN, T. T., and HEIDELBERGER, C., *In vitro* malignant transformation of mouse prostate cells with carcinogenic hydrocarbons. *Proc. Amer. Ass. Cancer Res.*, **9**, 13 (1968).

CHEN, T. T., and HEIDELBERGER, C., The cultivation *in vitro* of cells derived from adult C3H mouse ventral prostate. *J. nat. Cancer Inst.* in press (1969a).

CHEN, T. T., and HEIDELBERGER, C., Malignant transformation of mouse prostate cells *in vitro* by 3-methylcholanthrene. *J. nat. Cancer Inst.*, in press (1969b).

DIPAOLO, J. A., and DONOVAN, P. M., Properties of Syrian hamster cells transformed in the presence of carcinogenic hydrocarbons. *Exp. Cell Res.*, **48**, 361-377 (1967).

EAGLE, H., Amino acid metabolism in mammalian cell cultures, *Science*, **130**, 432-437 (1959).

GIOVANELLA, B. C., and HEIDELBERGER, C., Biochemical and biological effects of heat on normal and neoplastic cells, *Proc. Amer. Ass. Cancer Res.*, **9**, 24 (1968).

GOSHMAN, L. M., and HEIDELBERGER, C., Binding of tritium-labeled polycyclic hydrocarbons to DNA of mouse skin. *Cancer Res.*, **27**, 1678-1688 (1967).

HEIDELBERGER, C., Studies on the molecular and cellular mechanisms of hydrocarbon carcinogenesis. *J. cell. comp. Physiol.*, **64**, supplement 1, 129-148 (1964).

HEIDELBERGER, C., and GIOVANELLA, B. C., Studies on the molecular and cellular mechanisms of hydrocarbon carcinogenesis. *Adv. Biol. Skin*, **7**, 105-131 (1966).

HEIDELBERGER, C., and IYPE, P. T., Malignant transformation *in vitro* by carcinogenic hydrocarbons. *Science*, **155**, 214-217 (1967).

HEIDELBERGER, C., and IYPE, P. T., Malignant transformation *in vitro* with carcinogenic hydrocarbons. *In* H. Katsuta (ed.), *Cancer cells in culture*, pp. 351-363, Univ. of Tokyo Press, Tokyo (1968).

HOLLEY, R. W., and KIERNAN, J. A. "Contact inhibition" of cell division in 3T3 cells. *Proc. nat. Acad. Sci. (Wash.)*, **60**, 300-304 (1968).

HUBERMAN, E., and SACHS, L., Cell susceptibility to transformation and cytotoxicity by the carcinogenic hydrocarbon benzo(a)pyrene. *Proc. nat. Acad. Sci. (Wash.)*, **56**, 1123-1129 (1966).

KUROKI, T., and SATO, H., Transformation and neoplastic development *in vitro* of hamster embryonic cells by 4-nitroquinoline-1-oxide and its derivatives. *J. nat. Cancer Inst.*, **41**, 53-71 (1968).

LASNITZKI, I., Growth pattern of the mouse prostate gland in organ culture and its response to sex hormones, vitamins, and 3-methylcholanthrene. *Nat. Cancer Inst. Monograph 12, Biology of the prostate and related tissues*, pp. 381-403 (1963).

OSSOVSKI, L., and SACHS, L., Temperature sensitivity of polyoma virus, induction of cellular DNA synthesis and multiplication of transformed cells at high temperature. *Proc. nat. Acad. Sci. (Wash.)*, **58**, 1938-1943 (1967).

PREHN, R. T., A clonal selection theory of chemical carcinogenesis. *J. nat. Cancer Inst.*, **32**, 1-17 (1964).

PUCK, T. T., and MARCUS, P. I., A rapid method for viable cell titration and clone production with HeLa cells in tissue culture: the use of X-irradiated cells to supply conditioning factors. *Proc. nat. Acad. Sci. (Wash.)*, **41**, 432-447 (1955).

PUCK, T. T., MARCUS, P. I., and CIECIURA, S. J., Clonal growth of mammalian cells in vitro, growth characteristics of colonies from single HeLa cells with and without a "feeder" layer. *J. exp. Med.*, **103**, 273-284 (1956).

RÖLLER, M. R., and HEIDELBERGER, C., Attempts to produce carcinogenesis in organ cultures of mouse prostate with polycyclic hydrocarbons. *Int. J. Cancer*, **2**, 509-520 (1967).

SANDERS, F. K., and BURFORD, B. O., Morphological conversion of cells *in vitro* by N-nitrosomethylurea. *Nature (Lond.)*, **213**, 1171-1173 (1967).

SANFORD, K. K., "Spontaneous" neoplastic transformation of cells *in vitro*: Some facts and theories. *Nat. Cancer Inst. Monograph 26, Cell, tissue, and organ culture*, pp. 387-408 (1968).

TEMIN, H. M., Studies on carcinogenesis by avian sarcoma viruses. VI. Differential multiplication of uninfected and of converted cells in response to insulin. *J. cell. Physiol.*, **69**, 377-384 (1967).

41

Kei SATO,

Tadayuki SAITO and

Makoto ENOMOTO

Development of Sarcomas in Mice at Site of Injection with a New Carcinogen, Monoacetyl Derivative of 4-Hydroxyaminoquinoline

Acetylation of 4-hydroxyaminoquinoline 1-oxide (HAQO) yields a diacetyl derivative (DiAcHAQO) which, according to Kawazoe et al. [1], is the O,O'-diacetyl derivative. DiAcHAQO reacts readily with tissue nucleophiles such as DNA, sRNA, methionine, and albumin [2, 3]. On repeated administration to mice it induced high incidences of sarcomas at the site of injection and papillomas and carcinomas at the site of application to the skin [4, 5].

Recently Sato et al. [3] found that reduction of DiAcHAQO with H_2-Pd in ethyl ether yielded a compound (m.p. 180°) which appears to be a monoacetyl derivative of hydro-xyaminoquinoline (HAQ). This deduction is based on the molecular formula ($C_{11}H_{10}$ N_2O_2), the presence of an acetyl group as shown by infrared absorption data, and reducing activity with Tollen's reagent comparable to that of HAQO; 4-acetylaminoquinoline 1-oxide does not have reducing activity under these conditions. Furthermore, the infra-red spectrum of the new compound coincides with that of the monoacetyl derivative derived from authentic HAQ. Reduction of 4-nitroquinoline 1-oxide (NQO) with 3 moles of H_2 in the presence of acetic anhydride yielded the same product.

One O- or two N-monoacetyl derivatives of HAQ (I, II, II') are possible. Structure I is the most probable structure. The monoacetyl derivative does not give a ferric iron test for hydroxamic acids and the infra-red absorption of its acetyl group occurs at 1745 cm⁻¹. Upon the acetylation, the monoacetyl derivative gives a diacetyl derivative (III) (m.p. 138°). The infra-red absorption of its acetyl groups occurs at 1745 cm⁻¹ and 1640 cm⁻¹. By the catalytic reduction of the diacetyl derivative, a new monoacetyl derivative (IV) m.p.(140°) is obtained. The acetyl band of this monoacetyl derivative occurs at 1640 cm⁻¹, and the elemental analytical value of this compound coincides with that of acetylaminoquinoline ($C_{11}H_{10}N_2O$). However, the infra-red absorption data of authentic 4-acetylaminoquinoline (4AcAQ) (m.p. 171–173°) derived from 4-acetylaminoquinoline 1-oxide (4AcAQO) by catalytic reduction is not identical with that of the new compound (IV). The acetyl group of 4AcAQ and 4AcAQO shows a peak at 1670 cm⁻¹ and 1700 cm⁻¹, respectively. These findings suggest the following reaction process, providing conclusive evidence for determining the structure of those compounds related to HAQO [6].

We wish to report now on the carcinogenic activity of this monoacetyl derivative of HAQ (AcHAQ) and the comparison of its activity with that of DiAcHAQO. Female mice of the DDD strain (Institute of Medical Science, University of Tokyo), 5 weeks old and weighing about 20 g, were fed ad libitum a commercial pellet diet (CLEA (CE-2)) and tap water. The mice were injected subcutaneously in the right hind leg twice weekly for the first two weeks and once weekly for the following 16 weeks. Each injection consisted of 0.58 μmoles of compound in 0.1 ml of olive oil. The controls received the solvent alone.

AcHAQ induced sarcomas (diagnosed histologically as fibrosarcomas and myosarcomas) at the injection site in 17 of 20 mice (85%), and DiAcHAQO induced similar sarcomas in 13 of 21 mice (62%) (TABLE 1). The first sarcomas appeared at 2-1/2 and 3 months

*Wave number in IR spectrum.

after injection of AcHAQ and DiAcHAQO, respectively.

Both carcinogens induced ulceration or induration at the site of injection after administration of a few doses. Both compounds also caused systemic toxicity in some of the mice. Those mice dying from toxicity revealed cytotoxic changes in tissues with actively dividing cells (i.e., the mucosa of the small intestine, and the germ center of the lymph follicles in the spleen, lymph node, other lymph apparatus, and thymus).

The potent carcinogenicity of AcHAQ is also evident from the high incidence of subcutaneous sarcomas and lung adenomas which developed in DDD mice given a single subcutaneous injection of 53 mμmoles within 24 hours after birth (TABLE 2) [7].

Our data support the recent suggestion of Mori et al. [8, 9], that the N-oxide group may

TABLE 1

The induction of sarcomas by the subcutaneous injection of
NQO-derivatives into mice[1].

Compound injected	No. of injections[2]	No. of mice with sarcomas at injection site (period)	Effective no. of mice[3]	No. of mice that died tumor-free from toxicity (period)
AcHAQ	20	17 (84–200 days)	20	3 (1– 76 days)
DiAcHAQO	20	13 (102–207 days)	21	8 (9–128 days)
(vehicle only)	20	0	10	0

1) DDD, female; 5 wks.
2) 0.1 ml of olive oil containing 0.12 mg of AcHAQ or 0.15 mg of DiAcHAQO was injected subcutaneously twice (first two weeks) or once per week.
3) Based on the survival when the first tumor appeared.

43

TABLE 2

Tumor induction in DDD mice given a single subcutaneous injection of
each 53 mμmoles of NQO-derivatives within 24 hours after birth.

Compound	Total no. of mice injected	Early death (within 30 days)	Effective no. of mice[1]	No. of cases of			
				lung adenoma	subcutaneous sarcoma	leukemia or lymphosar- coma	others
Olive oil	34	9	20	1 (5.0)[2]	0 (0.0)	0 (0.0)	1[3]
4NQO	27	8	18	5 (27.8)	1 (5.5)	0 (0.0)	0
HAQO.HCl	31	16	13	6 (46.1)	6 (46.1)	3 (25.0)	0
AcAQO[4]	23	6	13	1 (7.7)	0 (0.0)	0 (0.0)	1[5]
DiAcHAQO	44	21	16	8 (50.0)	2 (12.5)	0 (0.0)	1[6]
AcHAQ	49	14	30	16 (53.3)	4 (13.3)	0 (0.0)	1[7]

1) Based on the survival when the first tumor appeared. All survival animals were killed on 400th days.
2) No. in parenthesis shows per cent of tumor cases against effective no. of mice.
3) Lymphogranuloma.
4) 4-acetylaminoquinoline-1-oxide.
5) Lymphoid tumor.
6) Embryonal carcinoma of the testis.
7) Adenocarcinoma of the mammary tissue.

not be essential for the carcinogenicity of NQO derivatives from their findings on the carcinogenicity of 2-nitroquinoline and 4-nitroquinoline. Furthermore, the greater carcinogenicity of our new monoacetyl derivative of HAQ as compared to that of 4-nitroquinoline suggests that AcHAQ might be a proximate carcinogen of 4-nitroquinoline. Yet, it is not certain that the conversion of AcHAQO to N-oxide compound *in vivo* is excluded. Further studies on this compound are in progress.

ACKNOWLEDGEMENT

This work was supported in part by the grant from the Ministry of Education, Japan. The authors wish to thank Drs. James A. Miller and Elizabeth C. Miller, McArdle Laboratory for Cancer Research, University of Wisconsin, Medical Center for their advice and a part of chemical analyses of the compound and also wish to thank Miss Keiko Miyata for her technical assistance.

44

References

[1] **Kawazoe, Y** and **Araki, M.:** Studies on chemical carcinogens. V. O, O'-diacetyl-4-hydroxyamino-quinoline 1-oxide. Gann, **58,** 485–487 (1967).

[2] **Enomoto, M., Sato, K., Miller, E. C.** and **Miller, J. A.:** Reactivity of the diacetyl derivative of the carcinogen 4-hydroxyaminoquinoline 1-oxide with DNA, RNA, and other nucleophiles. Life Sciences, **7,** 1025–1032 (1968).

[3] **Sato, K., Saito, T., Enomoto, M.** and **Saito, M.:** Chemical properties and carcinogenicity of the diacetyl derivatives of 4-hydroxyaminoquinoline 1-oxide. Proc. 28th Annual Meeting, Japanese Cancer Association, October, p.66 (1969). (in Japanese)

[4] **Enomoto, M., Miller, E. C.** and **Miller, J. A.:** Comparative carcinogenicity of 4-hydroxyaminoquino-line 1-oxide and its diacetyl derivative in mice and rats. Proc. Soc. Exptl. Biol. and Med., in press.

[5] **Kawazoe, Y., Araki, M.** and **Nakahara, W.:** Studies on chemical carcinogens. VIII. The structure -carcinogenicity relationship among derivatives of 4-nitro- and 4-hydroxyaminoquinoline 1-oxides. Chem. Pharm. Bull. (Tokyo), **17,** 544–549 (1969).

[6] **Enomoto, M., Sato, K., Miyata, K. Saito, T.** and **Saito, M.:** Comparative toxicities and carcinogeni-cities of NQO-derivatives. (I). In preparation.

[7] **Enomoto, M., Miyata, K., Saito, M., Sato, K.** and **Saito, T.:** Comparative study on toxicity and carcinogenicity of the various derivatives of 4-nitroquinoline 1-oxide in DDD mice. Proc. 29th Annual Meeting, Japanese Cancer Association, October, p.50 (1970). (in Japanese):

[8] **Mori, K., Kondo, M., Tamura, M., Ichimura, H.** and **Ohta, A.:** A new carcinogen, 2-nitroquino-line: Induction of lung cancer in mice. Gann, **60,** 609 (1969).

[9] **Mori, K., Kondo, M., Tamura, M., Ichimura, H.** and **Ohta, A.:** Induction of sarcoma in mice by a new carcinogen, 4-nitroquinoline. Gann, **60,** 663 (1969).

45

STUDIES ON THE MECHANISM OF 7,12-DIMETHYLBENZ[a] ANTHRACENE LEUKEMOGENESIS IN MICE
II. THE ROLE OF THYMUS IN DMBA LEUKEMOGENESIS*

HAYASE SHISA

Malignant lymphoma (lymphocytic leukemia) originating in the thymus can be induced at high incidence in mice when they are given a single injection of 7, 12-dimethylbenz[a]anthracene(DMBA) shortly after birth as summarized in our previous paper[1]. Development of both spontaneous and induced leukemias by viruses, chemicals, or X-ray irradiation is strongly influenced by the presence or absence of the thymus (reviewed by Miller 1962[2], Kaplan 1967[3]). The thymus may have two roles in murine leukemogenesis; first, the thymus provides the site of origin of leukemogenesis[4-9] and second, the thymus produces a humoral factor which is probably responsible for leukemia development[10].

The present report investigates the mechanism of DMBA leukemogenesis with reference to the role of the thymus, dealing with the following questions: (1) Whether the thymus is necessary for leukemia development when the baby mice are exposed to DMBA? (2) Whether thymectomy after DMBA exposure prevents leukemia development? (3) Whether reimplantation of the thymus restores the suscepti- bility of thymectomized animals to leukemia development? (4) The presence or absence of the thymus gives any influence on the phenotype of DMBA-induced leukemia?

Materials and Methods

Male and female Swiss mice, raised in our laboratory, were used. The method of DMBA in- jection, care of animals, check for tumor development, autopsy and histological observation were made the same as those described in our previous publication[1]. The experiments were composed

*This paper written in partial fulfilment of the requirements for the degree of Doctor of Medical Science of Mie Prefectural University School of Medicine.

of the following 3 major parts.

Experiment I. Baby mice were thymectomized at 3 days of age under the technique previously described[11]. Immediately after thymectomy, usually within less than 3 hours, they were given a single subcutaneous injection of 100 μg of DMBA. They were divided into 2 groups. One group of mice was grafted 7 days later with 1-day-old thymuses taken from non-injected Swiss mice of the same sex. Each animals received one whole thymus in the right inguinal fat pad. The other group of mice was inoculated intraperitoneally with two doses of 5–8 × 10⁶ viable spleen cells each on the 10th and 17th day of life. Pooled spleens (4–8 to a pool) of adult non-treated Swiss mice, aged about 10 weeks old, were finely minced with scissors, then suspended in sterile cold physiological saline. The cell suspensions were passed through a glass filter with the pore size of 100–120 μ. Trypan blue staining revealed that more than 90% of cells thus prepared were viable. This experiment was terminated at 8 months after birth.

Experiment II. The effect of thymectomy and of thymusgrafting into thymectomized animals on leukemogenesis in neonatally DMBA-treated Swiss mice was studied. Newborns that were given a single subcutaneous injection of 60 μg of DMBA were subjected to either thymectomy or sham-thymectomy at the age of 20±1 or 35±2 days. About half of the mice thymectomized at 35 days were grafted subcutaneously with 1-day-old Swiss thymus or with autochthonous thymus immediately after thymectomy.

Experiment III. The thymuses taken from 20-day-old or 35-day-old Swiss mice injected with DMBA at birth were transplanted subcutaneously into intact or thymectomized Swiss mice to investigate the presence of autonomous leukemia cells in the thymus. Intact 2-day-old Swiss mice were inoculated intraperitoneally with about 10⁷ viable thymus cells which were made from 7 pooled thymuses of 35-day-old Swiss mice given DMBA at birth.

Results

I. Leukemia development after injection of 7,12-dimethylbenz[a]anthracene in thymectomized mice.

As illustrated in Table 1, the leukemia incidence in intact Swiss mice of our colony was 3.7%, 5 out of 134 mice, at the age of 8 months. A single injection of 100 μg of DMBA on the 3rd day of life caused a marked increase in the incidence of leukemia; 80.6%, 29 out of 36 mice. Thus induced leukemias were the thymic lymphocytic lymphomas. Thymectomy performed on the 3rd day of life did not yield any severe wasting syndrome in Swiss mice. The incidence of leukemia in thymectomized mice was 2.0%, 2 out of 100 mice. However, when DMBA was given concomitantly at a doses of 100 μg after thymectomy, almost all animals (16 out of 20 mice) died within 10 weeks after DMBA injection of a cachectic lethal condition probably due to profound immunologic defects. In this group, only one of 4 surviving animals developed myeloid leukemia. Both grafting of 1-day-old thymus and intraperitoneal injection of spleen cells were capable of repairing immunological deficiency of thymectomized, DMBA-treated mice, and 40 out of

47

Table 1

Leukemia Development after Injection of 7,12-dimethylbenz[a]anthracene
in Thymectomized Swiss Mice.

Treatment			No. of mice at start of treatment	No. of mice at 10 weeks of age	Mice with leukemia***			
Thymec-tomy*	DMBA injection**	Others			Lymphocytic	Myeloid and others	Total (%)	Average age (Days)
−	−	−	−	134	4	1	5(3.7)	168.4
−	+	−	41	36	28	1	29(80.6)	107.5
+	−	−	113	100	0	2	2(2.0)	185.0
+	+	−	20	4	0	1	1(25.0)	168.0
+	+	Thymus# grafting	24	13	4(3)*ᵃ	1	5(38.5)	176.5
+	+	Spleen cell## inoculation	36	27	0	7	7(25.9)	157.5

*Thymectomy on the 3rd day of life. **100 μg of DMBA was injected subcutaneously at 3rd day of life (3 hours after thymectomy). ***Observation period : 8 months after birth. *ᵃ In parenthesis : Grafted thymus were involved in 3 leukemic mice. #Non-treated 1-day-old thymuses were grafted on the 10th day of life. ##Two doses of 5–8 × 10⁶ spleen cells of non-treated adult Swiss mice were inoculated intraperitoneally on the 10th and 17th day of life, respectively.

60 mice survived over 10 weeks of age. However, no apparent increase in the incidence of leukemia was observed. In the group of thymusgrafting, three leukemias with the involvement of implanted thymus, one non-thymic lymphoma and one myeloid leukemia developed. Among 36 mice injected with spleen cells, 7 mice developed leukemias which were non-thymic type lymphomas.

II. Effects of thymus grafting on leukemia development in thymectomized mice given 7,12-dimethylbenz[a]anthracene at birth.

As seen in Table 2, 84 per cent of the mice that received an injection of 60 μg of DMBA at birth developed thymic leukemia within 6 months after the injection. Thymectomy on the 20th day and 35th day of life reduced the incidence of leukemia to 20.8%, 5 out of 24 mice and 21.7%, 10 out of 46 mice, respectively. No restoration of leukemia incidence was observed in the DMBA-treated thymectomized mice by reimplantation of either 1-day-old isogenic thymus or autochthonous thymuses. To exclude the possibility that failure of restoration was mainly based upon early rejection of the grafts due to non-homogeneity of Swiss mice, recovery assay of the thymus grafts placed in the subcutaneous site was carried out in various designs as illustrated in Table 3. This assay demonstrated that recovery rates were over 75% in all the experimental groups tested. Histologic study revealed that grafted thymuses showed the normal architecture.

In experiments I and II, morphological difference was noticed between leukemias occurring in thymectomized mice and those developing in thymectomized

48

Table 2

Leukemia Development in Thymectomized Swiss Mice Given 60 μg
of 7,12-dimethylbenz[a]anthracene within 24 Hours after Birth.

Treatments		No. of mice used**	Mice with leukemia****			
Thymectomy	Thymus grafting*		6M***	6–8M	Total (%)	Average age (days)
—	—	75	63	0	63(84.0)	113.6
at 20 days of age	—	24	1	4	5(20.8)	271.0
at 35 days of age	—	46	9	1	10(21.7)	144.8
at 35 days of age	1-day-old# thymuses	34	4(3)*ᵃ	6(4)	10(29.4)	195.9
at 35 days of age	Autochthonous## thymuses	24	2(2)	2(2)	4(16.6)	183.0

*Thymus grafting was performed immediately after thymectomy at 35 days of age in the right inguinal fat pad. **Number of mice which survived over 60 days. ***Observation period ; 6 months after DMBA injection. ****Observation period ; 8 months after DMBA injection. *ᵃ In parenthesis : Number of leukemic mice with enlarged grafted thymus. #1-day-old thymuses of non-treated Swiss mice. ##Removed thymuses at 35-day-old immediately placed into the right inguinal fat pad of the same animals.

Table 3

Recovery of Thymus Grafts 21 Days after Subcutaneous
Transplantation in Swiss Mice.

Recipient		Age of** thymus grafts	No. of** grafted thymuses	Weight of recovered thymuses			Percentage of recovery (>15mg)
Age	Thymectomy*			<15 mg	15–20mg	20mg<	
35 days	—	1-day-old	21	3	2	16	85.7
35 days	+	1-day-old	17	4	3	10	76.5
35 days#	+	1-day-old	24	4	4	16	83.3
35 days	+	35-day-old##	12	0	1	11	100.0

*Thymectomy at 35 days of life. **Grafted thymus of the same sex was placed in the right inguinal fat pad. #Recipients were given 60 μg of DMBA at birth. ##Thymus grafts from autochthonous hosts.

mice with thymus grafts. Gross examination indicated that leukemias in thymecto-mized animals showed moderate or marked enlargement of lymph nodes and spleen, frequently associated with hepatomegaly. In the cases of leukemias developing in thymectomized mice with thymus grafts, enlargement of the *subcutaneous* thymus was usually the first sign of leukemia development, and occasionally this was the only symptom of leukemia at autopsy (Fig. 1). Of couse, some cases were accom-panied by enlargement of lymph nodes and hepatosplenomegaly. Histologically, leukemias appearing in the mice with thymus grafts were essentially lymphocytic. Leukemic involvement of grafted thymus was characterized by marked accumula-

49

tion of lymphocytic leukemic cells which had the same cytological characteristics as that of leukemic cells of thymic lymphomas developing in DMBA-treated, sham-thymectomized mice (Fig. 2). Leukemias found in the mice without thymus were composed of cells with those characteristics; undifferentiated type leukemias. Leukemic cells were generally larger than lymphocytic leukemia cells and were polygonal, well-defined forms possessing an ample cytoplasm that surrounds an oval, sharply outlined nucleus in which the chromatin is rich and evenly distributed. The cell had a tendency to aggregate and to show nodular infiltration. Such morphological difference was most clearly recognized in the foci of leukemic infiltration into the liver (Figs. 3, 4).

Table 4
Transplantation Assay of Thymuses of 7,12-dimethylbenz[a]anthracene
Treated Swiss Mice for the Presence of Leukemic Cells*

Age of thymuses transplanted	Number of thymuses transplanted	Number of** recipients	Mice with transplanted leukemia		
			Number	(%)	Average latency (Days)
20 days	16	9	0	0	—
35 days	58	58	3	5.2	85.0
35 days	32	32*	2	6.3	56.0
35 days	7**	7**	0	0	—

*Thymuses used for transplantation assay were taken from mice given 60 μg of DMBA within 24 hours after birth. **Each recipients received grafting of 1 or 2 thymuses at 35±2 days after birth. ‡Recipients were thymectomized prior to thymus transplantation. ‡‡Thymus cell suspension was made from 7 pooled thymuses and 10^7 viable cells were given intraperitoneally into intact 2-day-old Swiss mice.

III. Transplantation assay of thymuses of 7,12-dimethylbenz[a]anthracene treated mice for the presence of autonomous leukemia cells.

The thymuses taken from 20-day-old or 35-day-old Swiss mice injected with DMBA at birth were transplanted subcutaneously into intact or thymectomized Swiss mice (Table 4). None of 16 thymuses from 20-day-old mice and only 3 out of 58 thymuses from 35-day-old mice (5.2%) produced local tumors or generalized leukemias within 100 days after transplantation. Similarly, transplantation assay with thymectomized recipients was positive in only 2 out of 32 thymuses of the same age (6.3%). Intraperitoneal inoculation of thymus cell suspension gave negative results.

Discussion

The present experiments demonstrated that the incidence of leukemia evoked by DMBA in Swiss mice which were thymectomized either before or after DMBA-treatment fell into range of 20–30% in all experimental groups; namely that Swiss mice were less susceptible to DMBA-leukemogenesis when their thymuses were removed. Leukemia developed in about 30% in the thymectomized mice even when they received thymus-grafting 7 days after DMBA exposure, suggesting that leukemogenic action of DMBA is short-lasting, and neoplastic transformation of target cells may take place shortly after DMBA injection. Marked prevention of leukemia development was attained by thymectomy performed at 20 or 35 days after DMBA exposure. 35-day-old thymuses of neonatally DMBA-treated mice as shown in transplantation assay, had inadequate quantity of autonomous leukemic cells to produce transplantable leukemia in new intact hosts. Although it can be accepted that the thymus contains the cells most susceptible to DMBA, a possibility that other hematopoietic tissues such as bone marrow harbor target cells which migrate after neoplastic transformation into the thymus and form a tumor[12] there remains to be studied. This means in turn that the thymus provides the most favourable site for proliferation of leukemic cells which underwent neoplastic transformation outside the thymus. This possibility may be further supported by the fact that the direct injection of 20 μg of DMBA into the thymus of 30-day-old Swiss mice resulted in a very low leukemia incidence (2 out of 25 mice)[13]. But this result disagrees with that of the several investigators[14,15]. The incidence of chromosomal aberrations evoked by DMBA in cells of hematopoietic orgnas appears to be correlated to the incidence of DMBA lymphoma[16]; population of the target cells to DMBA may be correlated to frequency of DMBA leukemias. Bone marrow cells were most susceptible to the incidence of chromosomal aberration and thymus cells were one-tenth less susceptible than those of the bone marrow. The inhibitory effect of thymectomy was not reversed by reimplantation of neonatal or autochthonous thymuses. This is the same as that found in urethan leukemogenesis[17], but in contrast to reversal in 20-methylcholanthrene[18] and in radiation leukemogenesis[19]. Radiation leukemogenesis is proved to be mediated by the leukemia virus[20]. Aside from the question whether or not leukemogenic action of DMBA is mediated by virus, there is no exact explanation to account for such a significant difference in restoring effect of thymus implantation. The assumption that the action of urethan on the thymus is direct, whereas that of radiation is indirect[17] could be possibly applied to DMBA leukemogenesis. It is also possible that the subcutaneous thymus grafts might be an inadequate site for proliferation of the DMBA-induced leukemic cells. But we need further analysis.

It should be emphasized that a difference in histopathologic patterns was observed between leukemias developing in thymectomized hosts and those occurring in thymectomized hosts with thymus grafts. Large leukemic cells in thymectomized

51

hosts appear to be in an undifferentiated stage. In the hosts that were thymectomized before or after DMBA injection and then received thymus grafts, possibly
leukemic cells infiltrated primarily into the grafted thymus in many cases resulting in its marked enlargement with a tendency towards lymphocytic maturation.
It is common in both experiments presented in Tables I and II that thymus
grafting did not augment the leukemia incidence in thymectomized hosts, but
resulted in the cytological changes of leukemic cells. This may indicate that
lymphocytic maturation of leukemic cells is controlled by the function of the thymus:
determination of the phenotype of leukemia as lymphocytic (or lymphoblastic)
leukemia or lymphosarcoma is strongly influenced by the presence of the thymus.
Whether this is mediated by the systemic action of the lymphocytosis stimulating
factor[10,21] or whether this is due to the tissue environment of the thymus into which
leukemic cells migrate, await a solution. This hypothesis can account for the
almost complete inhibition of lymphocytic leukemia development in thymectomized
AKR mice[11,22].

Summary

DMBA-induced leukemias are essentially of thymic lymphocytic leukemia.
Incidence of lymphocytic leukemia in the Swiss mice that received thymectomy
before DMBA injection was reduced. A few leukemia other than lymphocytic
leukemia developed in the DMBA-treated Swiss mice that were either grafted with
thymus or injected with spleen cells after thymectomy. Thymectomy performed
after DMBA injection also markedly reduced the leukemia development. Grafting
of the thymuses, isogenic or autochthonous, had no restoring effect on the leukemia
incidence in thymectomized mice. Morphological difference was observed between leukemias developing in thymectomized mice and those developing in animals
thymectomized and receiving thymus grafts. This suggests that the thymus has
a capacity of inducing the lymphocytic maturation of leukemic cells.

Acknowledgement

I wish to express my sincere gratitude to Dr. Yasuaki Nishizuka and Dr. Kazuya
Nakakuki for their many helpful suggestions and their continuing interests and
supports. I acknowledge also technical assistance of Mrs. Hiromi Tanabe and
Miss Natsue Aoki. This investigation was supported in part by a Grant-in-aid
for Scientific Research from the Ministry of Education of Japan and a Grant from
the Anna Fuller Fund, Conn., U.S.A., which are gratefully acknowledged.

References

1) Shisa, H., Mie Med. J., **19** (1969) 89.

2) Miller, J.F.A.P., Adv. Cancer Res., **6** (1962) 291.

3) Kaplan, H.S., Cancer Res., **27** (1967) 1325.

4) Dann, T.B., Moloney, J.B., Green, A.W., Arnold, B., J. Nat. Cancer Inst. **26** (1961) 189.

5) Rappaport, H., Baroni, C., Cancer Res., **22** (1962) 1067.

6) Goodman, S.B., Block., M.H., Cancer Res., **23** (1963) 1634.

7) Siegler, R., Rich, M.A., Cancer Res., **24** (1964) 1406.

8) Metcalf, D., J. Nat. Cancer Inst., **37** (1966) 425.

9) Siegler, R., Harrell, W., Rich, M.A., J. Nat. Cancer Inst., **37** (1966) 105.

10) Metcalf, D., Ann. N.Y. Acad. Sci., **73** (1958) 113.

11) Nakakuki, K., Shisa, H., Nishizuka, Y., Acta Haem., **38** (1967) 317.

12) Ball, J.K., J. Nat. Cancer Inst., **41** (1968) 553.

13) Shisa, H., Nishizuka, Y., (unpublished data).

14) Rask-Nielsen, R., J. Nat. Cancer Inst., **16** (1956) 1129.

15) Chieco-Bianchi, L., Fiore-Donati, L., Tridente, G., De Benedictis, G., Tumori, **51** (1965) 53.

16) Kurita, Y., Shisa, H., Matsuyama, M., Nishizuka, Y., Tanaka, R., Yoshida, T.H., Gann, **60** (1969) 91.

17) Berenblum, I., Bioato, L., Trainin, N., Cancer Res., **26** (1966) 361.

18) Law, L.W., Miller, J.H., J. Nat. Cancer Inst., **11** (1950) 425.

19) Kaplan, H.S., Brown, M.S., Paull, J., Cancer Res., **13** (1953) 677.

20) Lieberman, M., Kaplan, H.S., Science, **130** (1959) 387.

21) Hand, T., Caster, R., Luckey, T.D., Biochem. Biophys. Res. Comm., **26** (1967) 18.

22) Nakakuki, K., Nishizuka Y., Gann, **55** (1964) 509.

1. Enlargement of thymus graft (arrow) in a DMBA-treated male Swiss mouse that was thymectomized at 35 days of age and then grafted with 1-day-old Swiss male thymus.
2. Leukemic involvement of transplanted thymus of the same mouse shown in Fig. 1. Note leukemic cells with typical lymphocytic morphology. H.E., × 290.
3. Leukemic infiltration in the liver of a 139-day-old Swiss mouse that was given DMBA at birth and then thymectomized at 35 days of life. Note aggregated undifferentiated large and polygonal tumor cells with a oval sharply outlined nucleus in which the chromatin is rich and evenly distributed. H.E., × 450.
4. Leukemic infiltration in the liver of a 158-day-old Swiss mouse that was given DMBA at birth and thymectomized and then grafted with own thymus subcutaneously at 35 days of life. Note diffuse colonization by leukemic cells with morphological characteristics of the lymphocytic type. H.E., × 450.

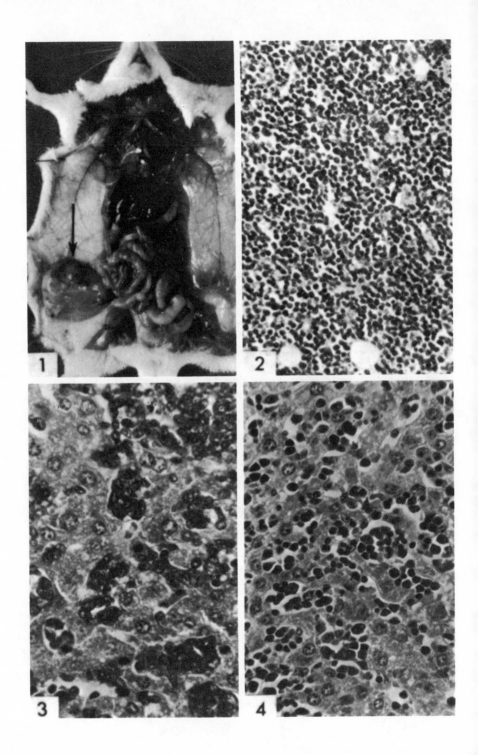

OOCYTE DESTRUCTION AND OVARIAN TUMORIGENESIS
AFTER DIRECT APPLICATION OF A CHEMICAL CARCINOGEN
(9:10-DIMETHYL-1:2-BENZANTHRACENE) TO THE MOUSE OVARY

by

Torben KRARUP

Ovarian tumours in mice can be induced by different methods: X-irradiation (Furth and Butterworth, 1936; Guthrie, 1958), transplantation of an ovary into the spleen (Biskind and Biskind, 1944 (rats); Guthrie, 1957) or into other organs of a gonadectomized host (Guthrie, 1959), application of a carcinogenic hydrocarbon either externally (Howell et al., 1954; Marchant, 1957; Mody, 1960) or internally (Biancifiori et al., 1961; Krarup, 1967) or genetic deletion of germ cells (Russell and Fekete, 1958; Murphy and Russell, 1963). The latency period depends on the experimental method and the strain of mice used.

Cellular changes begin to develop early during the latent period and lead ultimately to neoplastic growth. Probably the most important cellular event in the ovaries is the destruction of oocytes. After X-irradiation oocyte destruction begins immediately and is accomplished before tumour growth takes place (Guthrie, 1958;

55

Peters, 1969). Disappearance of follicles has been reported to occur in intrasplenic ovaries early after the transplantation operation (Guthrie, 1957), and the ultimate intrasplenic ovarian tumours contain no follicles (Biskind and Biskind, 1944). A reduction in the number of all sizes of follicles is already seen 1 month after treatment with a chemical carcinogen (Marchant, 1957), and normal follicles are seldom seen after the appearance of tumour nodules in the ovaries (Kuwahara, 1967). The number of small oocytes was reduced within one or two weeks after application of a chemical carcinogen—regardless of whether the carcinogen was given by mouth, intraperitoneally, or painted directly on to the ovaries (Krarup, 1967). It was suggested that the early destruction of oocytes plays an important role in the subsequent development of ovarian tumours. This is supported by the observation that a genetically early deletion of oocytes invariably results in ovarian tumours (Russell and Fekete, 1958; Murphy and Russell, 1963).

This paper reports on the effect of a single direct application of a carcinogenic hydrocarbon to the surface of the ovaries on the oocyte response and the subsequent pathological ovarian changes.

MATERIAL AND METHODS

Mice of the Street strain were used.

For application the chemical carcinogen 9:10-dimethyl-1:2-benzanthracene, (DMBA, obtained from Fluka AG, Chemische Fabrik, Buchs, SG, Switzerland) was prepared as a 0.5% solution in olive oil.

Thirty-five female mice aged 21 days were anaesthetized with ether, and both ovaries were exposed through lumbo-dorsal incisions. The ovaries were pulled out into the operating field by grasping the periovarian fat pad with a small forceps. The surface of the ovaries was painted with the DMBA-solution by means of a cotton swab. After painting, the wounds were sutured. Five of the mice were repainted after one week (at the age of 28 days) and 2 of these had a third painting after another week (at the age of 35 days).

Nine mice of the same age were used as controls; their ovaries were painted with olive oil using the same technique. Twenty untreated mice represented a second control group.

The animals were housed 3 to 5 mice to a cage until sacrifice. They were killed and their ovaries examined at different age intervals (Table I). The ovaries were fixed in Bouin's solution, embedded in paraffin, and serial sections at 5μ were stained with haematoxylin and eosin.

The ovarian pathology was studied, and differential oocyte counts were performed.

The oocytes were divided into two main groups: 1) the small oocytes, i.e. $20\,\mu$ or less in diameter, 2) the growing and large oocytes, i.e. those germ cells that have begun to grow and have a diameter of more than $20\,\mu$, as well as those that have reached their maximum diameter of $70\,\mu$ (Peters and Levy, 1964).

The small oocytes were counted in every tenth section, and the growing and large oocytes were counted in every fifth section using the nucleolus

TABLE I

NUMBER AND AGE OF MICE IN CONTROL AND EXPERIMENTAL GROUPS

Age at sacrifice	Untreated controls	Painted with olive oil	Painted once with DMBA	Painted twice with DMBA	Painted three times with DMBA
22 days	2		5		
28 days	2	2	3		
35 days	2		3		
42 days	2		2		
49 days	2		2	3	2
3 months . . .	2		3		
6 months . . .	2	3	4		
9 months . . .	2	2	4		
12 months . . .	4	2	4		

TABLE II

NUMBER OF OOCYTES IN OVARIES OF UNTREATED CONTROL MICE

Age of mice		Small oocytes	Growing and large oocytes	Total oocytes	$\frac{\text{Growing and large}}{\text{total}} \times 100(\%)$
22 days		3657	521	4178	
		3214	525	3739	
	Average	3435	523	3958	13
28 days		2510	378	2888	
		3105	360	3465	
	Average	2807	369	3176	12
35 days		2843	121	2964	
		3228	239	3467	
	Average	3035	180	3215	6
42 days		3070	264	3334	
		2550	171	2721	
	Average	2810	217	3037	7
49 days		2470	221	2691	
		1801	396	2197	
	Average	2135	309	2444	13
3 months		2457	625	3082	
		1828	407	2235	
	Average	2142	516	2658	19
6 months		1057	493	1550	
		838	500	1338	
	Average	947	496	1444	34
9 months		671	310	981	
		250	278	528	
	Average	460	294	754	39
12 months		179	128	307	
		286	100	386	
		343	61	404	
		214	50	264	
	Average	255	85	340	25

as marker. The total number of oocytes in one ovary was calculated by the method described by Peters and Levy (1964).

Oocyte counts of the untreated controls were done only in one ovary of each animal, as Jones (1957) found no difference between the two ovaries of several strains of mice. In the DMBA-treated mice, however, as well as in the olive oil controls, counts were performed on both ovaries of all mice older than 3 months, as the pathological development sometimes differed in the two ovaries.

RESULTS

Oocyte counts

Ovaries of untreated control mice

The number of oocytes present in normal ovaries of mice between the ages of 3 weeks and

12 months was determined in 20 animals (Table II, Fig. 1).

At the age of 22 days one ovary contains about 3,400 small oocytes; this number is halved within the next 9 weeks. After the age of 3 months a more gradual elimination occurs. About 250 small oocytes still reside in one ovary of a 1-year-old animal. The number of growing and large oocytes, however, decreases in number between the 22nd and the 35th days of life to reach a minimum that lasts for the next 2 weeks. Then a rapid increase occurs, reflecting the onset of fertile life of the animals. After the age of 6 months a gradual elimination of the growing and large oocytes occurs.

Ovaries painted with olive oil

The number of oocytes present in ovaries at different time intervals after painting with olive oil was determined in 9 mice (Table III, Fig. 1).

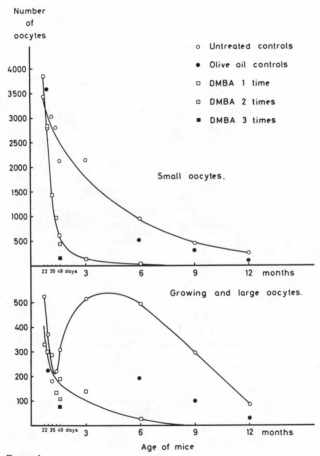

FIGURE 1
Number of small oocytes and of growing and large oocytes in ovaries of control mice and experimental mice in relation to age.

58

At the age of 28 days (i.e. one week after painting) the number of oocytes was found to be the same as in the untreated controls (the difference is not significant, P>0.1). However, at the age of 6, 9, and 12 months the number of small oocytes as well as of growing and large oocytes was significantly reduced (small oocytes: P<0.01; growing and large oocytes: P<0.02 at the age of 12 months).

Ovaries painted once with DMBA

The oocyte number remaining in one or both ovaries at different ages after one application of DMBA was investigated in 30 animals (Table IV, Fig. 1).

A reduction in the number of small oocytes is initiated within the first two weeks after the treatment. At the age of 35 days the reduction of the number of oocytes is suggestive but not statistically significant (P>0.05), however, a week later the oocyte number is definitely reduced (P<0.05). The rapid reduction of small oocytes continues up to the age of 49 days after which time a more gradual elimination sets in. Both ovaries of each

mouse aged 3, 6, 9, and 12 months were examined, and it appears from the individual counts (Table IV) that total depletion of small oocytes may already be present at the age of 3 months; at the age of 9 months only one ovary out of eight still contained a few small oocytes.

A decrease in the number of growing and large oocytes, comparable to that seen in the untreated controls, was found within the first 3 weeks after treatment; after this time the decrease of the growing and large oocytes continued gradually until complete exhaustion of oocytes occurred between the ages of 6 and 9 months. There was no increase in the number of growing and large oocytes at the time of onset of sexual maturity.

Ovaries painted 2 or 3 times with DMBA

The number of oocytes remaining in the ovaries of animals that were painted with DMBA more than once was determined in 5 mice, when they had reached the age of 49 days (Table V).

Though the results are not statistically significant (P>0.3) they seem to suggest that multiple painting hastens the oocyte destruction (Fig. 1).

TABLE III

NUMBER OF OOCYTES IN OVARIES PAINTED WITH OLIVE OIL

Age of mice	Mouse number		Small oocytes		Growing and large oocytes		Total oocytes		$\dfrac{\text{Growing and large}}{\text{total}} \times 100(\%)$
28 days . . .	x-12		3520		189		3709		
	x-13		3650		254		3904		
		Average	3585		222		3807		6
6 months . .	x-33		529	207	275	118	804	325	
	x-36		557	378	289	114	846	492	
	x-38		900	1	171	1	1071	1	
		Average	514		193		707		27
9 months . .	x-55		86	171	107	89	193	260	
	x-63		500	464	96	100	596	564	
		Average	305		98		403		24
12 months . .	x-115		71	164	21	46	92	210	
	x-122		71	57	25	32	96	89	
		Average	91		31		122		25

[1] Ovary lost during technical processing.

TABLE IV

NUMBER OF OOCYTES IN OVARIES PAINTED ONCE WITH DMBA

Age of mice	Mouse number	Small oocytes		Growing and large oocytes		Total oocytes		$\frac{\text{Growing and large}}{\text{total}} \times 100(\%)$
22 days	x-1	3779		325		4104		
	x-2	5243		357		5600		
	x-3	4550		370		4920		
	x-4	2620		261		2881		
	x-5	3070		343		3413		
	Average	3852		331		4183		8
28 days	x-6	3070		369		3439		
	x-7	2900		254		3154		
	x-8	2520		275		2795		
	Average	2830		299		3129		10
35 days	x-14	1190		340		1530		
	x-15	613		272		885		
	x-16	2500		250		2750		
	Average	1434		287		1722		17
42 days	x-18	1080		129		1209		
	x-19	864		143		1007		
	Average	972		136		1108		12
49 days	x-23	242		158		400		
	x-24	980		221		1201		
	Average	611		189		800		24
3 months . . .	x-28	150	50	241	178	391	228	
	x-29	0	43	0	64	0	107	
	x-30	321	179	150	203	471	382	
	Average	124		139		263		53
6 months . . .	x-31	0	0	12	7	12	7	
	x-32	0	7	3	8	3	15	
	x-34	57	71	43	54	100	125	
	x-35	107	64	61	21	168	85	
	Average	38		26		64		41
9 months . . .	x-52	0	0	0	4	0	4	
	x-53	0	0	0	0	0	0	
	x-54	0	29	1	3	1	32	
	x-62	0	0	3	0	3	0	
	Average	4		1		5		20
12 months . . .	x-114	0	0	0	0	0	0	
	x-116	0	0	0	0	0	0	
	x-119	0	0	0	0	0	0	
	x-120	0	0	0	1	0	1	
	Average	0		0		0		

Ovaries of untreated control mice

The ovaries of normal mice at ages 22 days, 35 days, or 42 days were filled with oocytes and follicles. Small oocytes were found in groups and nests at the periphery of the ovaries; growing and large oocytes in varying stages of follicle development were distributed throughout most of the organ. Blood vessels in the periovarian capsule and capillaries in the outer ovarian cortex were rarely noted. In the youngest of the ovaries the amount of stroma was scant. However, at the ages of 35 to 42 days increasing amounts of stroma appeared, apparently originating from degenerating and degenerated follicles, which were found in increasing numbers from the 22nd to 42nd days of life.

be slightly luteinized in areas, but a diffuse luteinization of the whole stromal mass was never observed. In the ovaries of mice older than 6 months increasing amounts of cells with abundant vacuolated cytoplasm containing granules of brown pigment were noted. These pigmented cells could be found in groups or " corpora " as well as diffusely scattered among the stroma. Large amounts of stroma and pigmented cells were a prominent feature in the oldest ovaries. A few empty rings and pseudofollicles (Krarup, 1967) were occasionally found in 12-month-old ovaries.

The *senile ovaries* were thus composed of large amounts of stroma that was usually not luteinized. Pigmented cells and a few empty rings and pseudofollicles were characteristic structures; some follicles and corpora lutea were also present.

TABLE V

NUMBER OF OOCYTES IN OVARIES PAINTED 2 AND 3 TIMES WITH DMBA.
AGE OF MICE: 49 DAYS.

Painted	Mouse number	Small oocytes	Growing and large oocytes	Total oocytes	$\frac{\text{Growing and large}}{\text{total}} \times 100(\%)$
2 times	x-20	7	43	50	
	x-21	486	200	686	
	x-22	828	79	907	
	Average 440		107	547	20
3 times	x-26	86	39	125	
	x-27	200	107	307	
	Average 143		73	216	34

The first *corpora lutea* were found from the age of 35 or 42 days, and after that time, *i.e.* after onset of sexual maturity, *corpora lutea* of varying ages as well as different amounts of more or less luteinized stroma contributed to the structure of the ovary.

The normal ovaries of animals aged 7 weeks or more were thus composed of oocytes in various stages of follicle development and large fresh *corpora lutea* as well as older and smaller *corpora lutea*. Degenerating follicles as well as completely atretic follicles with a remnant of *zona pellucida* were likewise found at all ages. With advancing age the amount of stroma increased. This could

Ovaries painted with olive oil

The ovaries painted with olive oil were found to be morphologically normal at the age of 28 days (*i.e.* one week after painting). However, the ovaries of the 7 mice examined at ages between 6 months and one year revealed some abnormal features. These were most marked in the left ovary of mouse X-55 which, at the age of 9 months, showed the lowest number of oocytes (Table III).

The surface epithelium was thickened at 6 months and showed some tubular protrusions into the ovarian parenchyma at 9 and 12 months.

61

Empty rings could be found in the outer ovarian cortex at 6 months, and in the older animals pseudofollicles were also noted. Fresh and old *corpora lutea* were seen in 6-month-old ovaries. The ovaries of 9-month-old animals, however, showed only old *corpora lutea*, and the 1-year-old animals had no *corpora lutea*.

Follicles in all stages of development were seen at all ages though their number was reduced. Degenerating and atrophied follicles were found as in the normal ovaries.

In most of the ovaries at 6 and 9 months the amount of stroma was somewhat increased compared to the normal ovaries. The degree of luteinization of the stroma varied, but in some mice broad bands and large areas of luteinized stroma characterized the ovaries. However, the luteinization of the stroma became less prominent at the age of 12 months, at which age pigmented cells were found in large quantities.

Ovaries painted with DMBA

The ovaries that were painted with DMBA at the age of 21 days and examined 1 or 7 days later were characterized by marked periovarian hyperaemia and dilatation of capillaries in the outer cortical layer. Oocytes of all sizes were seen, but spaces in the subepithelial layer apparently left by degenerated small oocytes were characteristic. Follicle degeneration was marked, but probably not more extensive than in the control ovaries.

The first appearance of *corpora lutea* was noted in ovaries of 42-day-old mice, indicating the onset of sexual maturity, which thus proved not to be delayed.

Nevertheless the ovarian histology at 42 and 49 days was dominated by degenerative changes. This was the case whether the ovaries were painted one, two or three times with the carcinogen. The ovaries were somewhat smaller than normal. The surface epithelium was cuboidal and often double. Degeneration of follicles was a prominent feature, at this age more extensive than in the controls. Large amounts of stroma with areas of luteinization were characteristic. The luteinized stroma was apparently derived from degenerative follicular material (Fig. 2a and 2b). Occasionally an empty ring could be seen in the outer cortex.

At the age of 3 months most of the ovaries still contained oocytes in developing and large follicles. However, pathological changes were already present in all ovaries at this age *(potential preneoplastic changes)*. The surface epithelium was thickened and a concentration of dark-staining stroma cells was found beneath the surface epithelium. In the outer layer of the ovarian cortex empty rings and a few pseudofollicles were often found lying between the follicles and the *corpora lutea*. *Corpora lutea* of recent ovulation indicated by the presence of eggs in the tube, as well as old *corpora lutea* were seen. In some ovaries an accumulation of old *corpora lutea* seemed to be present, and the limit between adjacent *corpora lutea* was sometimes ill-defined. The amount of stroma was large; it was luteinized and formed bands and groups throughout the ovaries. Some degenerating follicles as well as

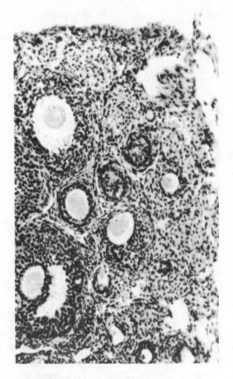

FIGURE 2a

Mouse x-18, 21 days after painting with DMBA. Degenerating follicles containing a shrunken oocyte. Groups of luteinized stroma cells. (× 100).

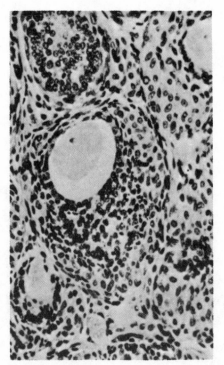

FIGURE 2b
Detail of Figure 2a. Luteinization in the wall of a degenerating follicle. (×250).

to make out whether a mass of lutein material was derived from degenerated follicles, and thus should be referred to as luteinized stroma, or whether it was formed from old *corpora lutea* that had merged together to form a diffuse mass of lutein material.

The lutein centre of the ovaries was surrounded by a rim of empty rings and pseudofollicles.

In most of the ovaries the surface epithelium had proliferated to form a few tubular protrusions into the ovarian parenchyma. Some pigmented cells were found in small groups among the lutein material. A few normal developing as well as large follicles were still present at this stage, although they no longer characterized the organs. Also some atrophied follicles with a

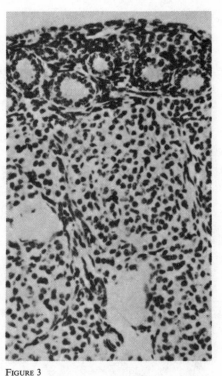

FIGURE 3
Mouse x-29, 3 months old. Potential preneoplastic ovary showing a rim of empty rings surrounding a centre of diffusely luteinized cell material. (×250).

many atretic follicles with a remnant of zona pellucida or a hyalinized ovum were present.

These changes were most prominent in the ovary of mouse X-29 (Fig. 3), that was depleted of oocytes at the age of 3 months (Table IV).

At the age of 6 months the potential preneoplastic changes had further progressed. The ovaries were now dominated by their lutein cell material. All of them showed an accumulation of old *corpora lutea*, some of which had merged together to form a diffuse mass of lutein tissue. Yet half of the ovaries showed signs of recent ovulation indicated by the presence of newly ruptured follicles and eggs in the tube. Large amounts of luteinized stroma were found throughout the ovaries contributing to the lutein structure. In many cases, however, it was no longer possible remnant of *zona pellucida* and a considerable number of hyalinized ova were present.

Unilateral ovarian tumours were found in 3 out of 4 mice at the age of 9 months. These were luteomas. The ovaries appeared yellow (as did the preneoplastic ones) and their size was equal to or slightly smaller than the size of control ovaries of comparable age ($2 \times 2 \times 2$ mm). The diagnosis of luteoma was thus solely based upon the microscopic structure of the organs. The cells were either arranged in small nodules (Fig. 4) or distributed diffusely without a specific pattern. They invaded the periovarian fat capsule (Fig. 5a and 5b) and showed some mitotic figures.

The surface epithelium formed downgrowths into the luteomas (Fig. 6). Patches of luteinized stroma could sometimes be recognized, and a

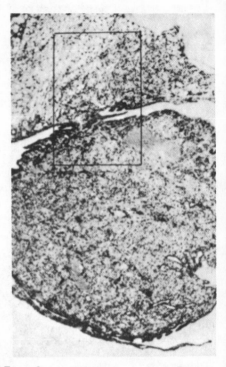

FIGURE 5a

Mouse x-116, 12 months old. Luteoma. The tumour cells have broken through the ovarian capsule and invade the periovarian fat. ($\times 40$).

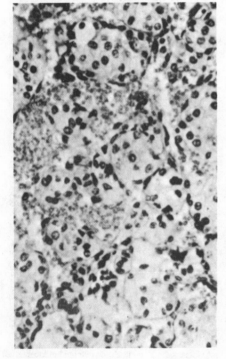

FIGURE 4

Mouse x-116, 12 months old. Luteoma consisting of nodules of luteoma cells. Interstitial bleeding. ($\times 250$).

few empty rings and pseudofollicles were found in some of the luteomas. Few pigmented cells were present.

In two mice the contralateral non-tumorous ovary showed preneoplastic changes as seen at earlier ages.

The contralateral non-tumorous ovary of the third mouse and both ovaries of the fourth mouse at this age had no follicles or *corpora lutea* and showed senile changes as described for old normal ovaries.

Ovarian tumours were found in the four 1-year-old mice.

One mouse had a luteoma in one ovary, while the contralateral ovary showed senile changes. Two mice had bilateral luteomas.

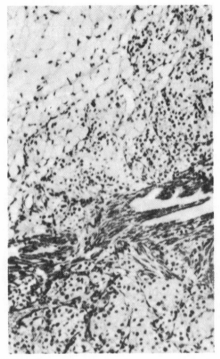

FIGURE 5b
Detail of Figure 5a. Tumour cells invading the peri-ovarian fat. (×100).

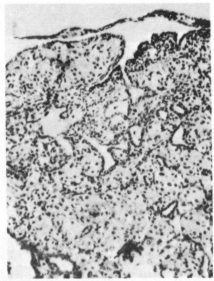

FIGURE 6
Mouse x-116, 12 months old. Nodular luteoma. The surface epithelium forms tubular protrusions into the luteoma tissue. (×100).

A 6 × 7 × 8 mm unilateral granulosa cell tumour was found in the fourth mouse at this age. Hormonal activity of this tumour was noted in the uterine endometrium, which showed signs of oestrogen stimulation (Fig. 7). The tumour cells had a striking resemblance to normal granulosa cells. They were mainly arranged in a follicular or nodular pattern, although areas of undifferentiated growth were found as well (Fig. 8a and 8b). Many mitotic figures suggested that the tissue was growing rapidly.

The contralateral ovary was small and atrophic. It was composed of a proliferative surface epithelium covering a broad cortical rim of pseudofollicles and empty rings. The ovarian centre contained small dark-staining stroma cells and large pigmented cells. Neither follicular nor luteal structures were found.

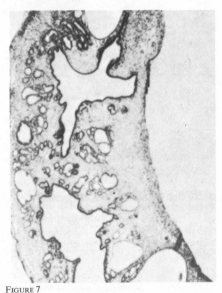

FIGURE 7
Mouse x-114, 12 months old. The endometrium of the uterus showing cystic hyperplasia. (×25).

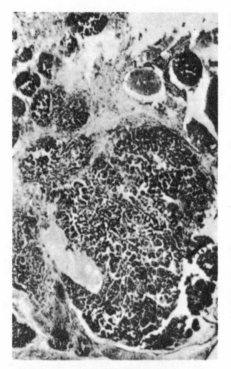

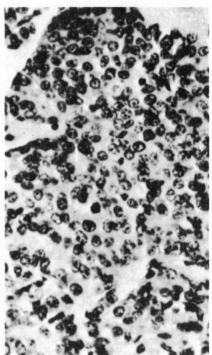

FIGURE 8a

Mouse x-114, 12 months old. Survey of granulosa cell tumour. Areas of undifferentiated growth as well as nodular or follicular patterns are seen. (×25).

FIGURE 8b

Mouse x-114, 12 months old. Granulosa cell tumour showing undifferentiated growth and some mitotic figures. (×400).

DISCUSSION

DMBA applied directly to the ovary affects the small oocytes and reduces their number within a short time (Krarup, 1967). This direct action of the chemical on the oocytes seems to be limited to the first 4 weeks after application. During this period the oocyte destruction rate is particularly high (Fig. 1), whereas after this time the small oocytes continue to be eliminated at a normal rate.

It thus appears that the small oocytes are the target cells. The growing and large oocytes are not affected by the carcinogen. Their elimination rate during the first 4 weeks after treatment is similar to that in the control ovaries, and is therefore considered to be physiological and cannot be attributed to an effect of the DMBA.

Why, then, is the complement of growing and large oocytes lower than normal throughout the maturity period of the animals (Fig. 1)? In the normal mice the number of growing and large oocytes, expressed as a percentage of the total number of oocytes, was found to increase with advancing age. This percentage proved to be about the same in the DMBA-treated mice (Table IV) as in the controls (Table II and Table III) at comparable ages, though their absolute number was reduced. The low number of growing and large oocytes may therefore be secondary to the reduction in the number of small oocytes.

The morphological development of the ovaries that follows the initial destruction of oocytes is not normal. The present material supports the observation (Krarup, 1967) that pathological changes develop in the ovaries while oocytes are still present; however, preneoplastic changes do not appear until the number of oocytes has been considerably reduced. The pathological development of the ovaries after treatment with the DMBA is secondary to the early oocyte destruction and apparently not caused by the DMBA directly. Development of ovarian tumours in mice is always preceded by destruction of oocytes. This is the case whether the induction is effected by X-irradiation (Guthrie, 1958; Peters, 1969) or intrasplenic ovary transplantation (Guthrie, 1957). Furthermore, mice born with only a few oocytes invariably develop ovarian tumours (Russell and Fekete, 1958; Murphy and Russell, 1963). There even seems to be a correlation between the rate of oocyte disappearence and the rate of pathological development: the faster the oocytes disappear, the earlier the pathological changes develop. One ovary painted with DMBA was already depleted of oocytes at the age of 3 months and that ovary showed more advanced preneoplastic changes than other ovaries of the same age which still contained oocytes.

The sequence of pathological events in the ovaries seems to follow a specific pattern. During the first stage large amounts of luteinized stroma are formed. This progresses to the stage of potential preneoplasia, during which *corpora lutea* persist, merge and form together with the luteinized stroma a diffuse mass of lutein material.

The further development can apparently follow different patterns, as different types of ovarian pathology were observed subsequent to the preneoplastic stage. These include: luteoma, granulosa cell tumour, or senile changes and atrophy. It is likely that the lutein material in the preneoplastic ovaries develops further and later forms the luteoma. The origin of the granulosa cell tumour, however, cannot be clarified from the present material. The development of a granulosa cell tumour within a preexisting luteoma was thought to occur after intrasplenic transplantation (Myhre, 1962) as well as after DMBA treatment (Mody, 1960), whereas the possibility of such a development was denied by Marchant (1957). Senile changes and atrophy of the ovary—not leading to tumour formation—could be the result of a regressive process in the preneoplastic ovaries.

The results of the olive oil control group showed that painting the ovaries with olive oil to some extent reduced the normal complement of oocytes at ages of 6, 9, and 12 months. This reduction proved to be statistically significant and as the ovarian structure also showed certain pathological features, the reduction caused by olive oil painting was considered to be real. It did not fall within the biological variation of the oocyte numbers, though this is known to be considerable for mice of the same strain and age (Jones and Krohn, 1961; Peters and Levy, 1964).

Intraperitoneal injection of olive oil, which for several months covers the surface of the ovaries, does not cause a reduction of the oocyte population (Krarup, unpublished data). It is therefore most likely that the insult to the ovaries was caused by the mechanical procedure, *i.e.* grasping the ovaries with a forceps, rather than by the oil on the ovarian surface. The mechanical trauma could be to the vessels of the ovaries. It is reported that experimental obstruction of ovarian vessels in rats later in life may cause ovarian dysfunction and even tumorigenesis (Fels, 1952; Fels, 1954).

The present study deals with the early effect of a carcinogenic hydrocarbon on mouse ovaries and the subsequent pathological development. Further studies are in progress to elucidate the relationship between the rate of oocyte disappearance and the rate of pathological development, to explore the morphological pathways in the late stages of ovarian tumorigenesis, and to investigate the reproductive competence of the ovaries during the process of oocyte disappearance.

ACKNOWLEDGEMENTS

The author wishes to thank Dr. Ema Levy for the painting of the ovaries.

BIANCIFIORI, C., BONSER, G. M., and CASHERA, F., Ovarian and mammary tumours in intact C_3Hb virgin mice following a limited dose of four carcinogenic chemicals. *Brit. J. Cancer*, 15, 270-283 (1961).

BISKIND, M. S., and BISKIND, G. S., Development of tumors in the rat ovary after transplantation into the spleen. *Proc. Soc. exp. Biol. (N.Y.)*, 55, 176-179 (1944).

FELS, E., Die Unterbindung des Ovarienstieles als Ursache anatomischer und funktioneller Genitalstörungen. *Arch. Gynäkol.*, 181, 380-390 (1952).

FELS, E., Effet de la ligature tubaire sur la fonction ovarienne chez le rat. *C. R. Soc. Biol. (Paris)*, 148, 1666 (1954).

FURTH, J., and BUTTERWORTH, J. S., Neoplastic diseases occurring among mice subjected to general irradiation with X-rays. *Amer. J. Cancer*, 28, 66-95 (1936).

GUTHRIE, M. J., Tumorigenesis in intrasplenic ovaries in mice. *Cancer*, 10, 190-203 (1957).

GUTHRIE, M. J., Tumorigenesis in ovaries of mice after X-irradiation. *Cancer*, 11, 1226-1235 (1958).

GUTHRIE, M. J., Tumourigenesis in ovaries of mice transplanted to the liver, kidney and adjacent tissues. *Nature (Lond.)*, 184, 916-917 (1959).

HOWELL, J. S., MARCHANT, J., and ORR, J. W., The induction of ovarian tumours in mice with 9:10-dimethyl-1:2-benzanthracene. *Brit. J. Cancer*, 8, 635-646 (1954).

JONES, E. C., *The aging ovary*. Thesis, University of Birmingham (1957).

JONES, E. C., and KROHN, P. L., The relationship between age, number of oocytes, and fertility in virgin and multiparous mice. *J. Endocrin.*, 21, 469-495 (1961).

KRARUP, T., 9:10-dimethyl-1:2-benzanthracene induced ovarian tumours in mice. *Acta path. microbiol. scand.*, 70, 241-248 (1967).

KUWAHARA, I., Experimental induction of ovarian tumours in mice treated with a single administration of 7,12-dimethylbenz(α)anthracene, and its histopathological observation. *Gann*, 58, 253-266 (1967).

MARCHANT, J., The chemical induction of ovarian tumours in mice. *Brit. J. Cancer*, 11, 452-464 (1957).

MODY, J. K., The action of four carcinogenic hydrocarbons on the ovaries of IF mice and the histogenesis of induced tumours. *Brit. J. Cancer*, 14, 256-266 (1960).

68

MURPHY, E. D., and RUSSELL, E. S., Ovarian tumorigenesis following genic deletion of germ cells in hybrid mice. *Acta Un. Int. Cancr.*, **19**, 779-782 (1963).

MYHRE, E., The histogenesis of granulosa cell tumours. An autoradiographic study of intrasplenic ovarian

transplants in gonadectomized rats. *Acta Un. Int. Cancr.*, **18**, 50-53 (1962).

PETERS, H., The effect of radiation in early life on the morphology and reproductive function of the mouse ovary, *in* Anne McLaren (ed.), *Advances in reproductive physiology*, Vol. 4, Logos Press, Ltd., London (in press).

PETERS, H., and LEVY, E., Effect of irradiation in infancy on the mouse ovary. *J. Reprod. Fertil.*, **7**, 37-45 (1964).

RUSSELL, E. S., and FEKETE, E., Analysis of W-series pleiotropism in the mouse: Effect of W^vW^v substitution on definitive germ cells and on ovarian tumorigenesis. *J. nat. Cancer Inst.*, **21**, 365-381 (1958).

THE INFLUENCE OF PRELIMINARY IRRITATION BY ACETIC ACID OR CROTON OIL ON SKIN TUMOUR PRODUCTION IN MICE AFTER A SINGLE APPLICATION OF DIMETHYL-BENZANTHRACENE, BENZOPYRENE, OR DIBENZ-ANTHRACENE

A. W. POUND

PREVIOUS studies (Pound and Withers, 1963; Pound, 1963, 1966) have shown that a single treatment of the skin of mice by scarification or chemical means, a short interval before a standard tumour-initiating treatment with urethane, augmented the yield of skin tumours. The augmenting effect was confined to the area affected by the preliminary treatment. The view advanced was that proliferating cells are more susceptible to the tumour-initiating action of urethane, since, when the preliminary treatment was made with croton oil, the number of tumours produced could be related to the cellular proliferation that occurred in the skin. In particular, it correlated with the number of cells replicating DNA at the time of injection of the urethane (Pound, 1966, 1968). The simplest hypothesis to explain these findings is that urethane acts during the replication of DNA. This may also be the case with the carcinogenic hydrocarbons (Pound, 1968).

This paper records the results of experiments to test the effect of preliminary irritation on the number of tumours produced by 3 carcinogenic hydrocarbons in single dosage without the use of a promoting treatment.

MATERIALS AND METHODS

Mice

Random bred male mice of the strain " Hall " (Pound, 1962) from the Department of Pathology at the Royal Brisbane Hospital were used. The animals were about 7 weeks of age and weighed 24–26 g. at the beginning of the experiments. They were housed in stainless steel compartments, each holding 10 mice, with a bed of coarse sawdust that was changed weekly, and were fed the diet previously used (Pound and Withers, 1963) supplied, with water, in excess of their needs. The animal house was air-conditioned at 22° C.

Chemicals

Acetic acid, Osta Chemical Company, analytical reagent. Acetone, By-Products and Chemicals Pty. Ltd., analytical reagent. Croton oil, Stafford, Allen & Sons, London. 7,12-dimethylbenz(a)anthracene (DMBA); benzo(a)pyrene

(BP); and dibenz(*a,h*)anthracene (DBA) were obtained from L. Light & Co., London, and were used without further purification.

The hair of the skin of the back of the mice was clipped with electric clippers immediately before applications to the skin, care being taken to avoid injury since, in the light of previous work (Pound and Withers, 1963), this alone might influence the tumour yields. It was also clipped before counting tumours when necessary.

The hydrocarbons were applied to the whole area of the skin of the back by painting with approximately 0·25 ml. of solutions of the compounds in acetone: 0·6%, 0·3%, 0·15% or 0·04% in the cases of BP and DMBA, and 0·3%, 0·15% or 0·04% in the case of DBA when the upper limit was defined by the solubility of the material. The area of skin covered was about 2·5 × 4·0 cm., that is about 10 sq. cm. The corresponding skin doses were therefore approximately 150, 75, 37, or 9 μg. per sq. cm. for BP and DMBA, and 75, 37, or 9 μg. per sq. cm. for DBA.

Experiments I, II and III

One thousand and eighty mice were distributed at random into compartments of 10. The compartments were arranged at random into 3 lots of 12 groups of 30 mice, i.e. 1 lot for each of the 3 hydrocarbons: Experiment I, DBA; Experiment II, BP; and Experiment III, DMBA.

For each experiment the mice were divided into 4 divisions, each comprising 3 groups of 30 mice. The mice in each division were given a preliminary application of 0·25 ml. of a 25% solution of acetic acid in acetone on the right side of the skin of the back, at 0, 24, 72 hours, or 9 days respectively before a single application of the carcinogenic hydrocarbon. The mice in the 3 groups of the 4 divisions were given an application of hydrocarbon to both sides of the skin of the back, 150, 37 or 9 μg. per sq. cm. for BP and DMBA and 75, 37 or 9 μg. per sq. cm. for DBA, respectively.

This gives a factorial arrangement in which the tumour yields on the 2 sides—treated and untreated with acetic acid—may be compared at 3 dose levels of the carcinogen and at 4 intervals of 0, 24, 72 hours and 9 days between the preliminary application of acetic acid and the application of the carcinogen. An interval of 0 hours between the 2 treatments means that the acetic acid solution was applied 15 minutes before the hydrocarbon, this being the time required for evaporation of the acetone solvent.

Experiment IV

Six hundred mice were divided at random into 3 lots of 200 and each lot divided into 5 groups of 40 mice.

The mice of 4 groups in each lot were given a preliminary application of 0·5 ml. of a 0·5% solution of croton oil in acetone to the whole area of the skin of the back at 0, 24, 72 hours and 9 days respectively, and the fifth group received no preliminary application, before the application of a carcinogenic hydrocarbon to the whole area of the skin of the back. The dose used was 75 μg. per sq. cm.

for all 3 hydrocarbons. One lot was treated with BP, the second lot with DMBA and the third lot with DBA.

Experiment V

Two control groups of 100 mice were painted once, one group with a 30 % solution of acetic acid in acetone, the other group with 0·5 % solution of croton oil in acetone. No carbinogenic hydrocarbons were administered.

The mice were examined at intervals for the presence of tumours in the treated area. A lesion was counted as a papilloma when it had reached a size of 1 mm. or more and persisted for 4 weeks or longer. A tumour was classified as malignant when it had grown progressively and had invaded the panniculus carnosus. Four sarcomata of the dermis developed in mice treated with the highest doses of DMBA but these are not included in the results. Malignant and doubtfully malignant growths were examined histologically but sections of clearly benign growths were not made. The number of tumours and their distribution on the skin of the back were recorded at fortnightly intervals, note being made of lesions that had regressed.

RESULTS

The application of croton oil or acetic acid in the amounts used leads promptly to acute inflammation in the skin. Epithelial hyperplasia soon begins and leads to keratin scaling from about the 4th or 5th day (Pound, 1968). In the control Experiment V, no tumours appeared during 40 weeks observation of the mice that had a single application of acetic acid (75 survivors) or croton oil (82 survivors). The natural incidence of skin papillomata in this strain of mouse at 12 months of age is less than one in a thousand over the whole area of the body (personal observation).

The smallest doses (9 μg. per sq. cm.) of the carcinogenic hydrocarbons did not produce any clinically obvious changes in the skin and did not alter the changes visible to the naked eye in areas previously treated with croton oil or acetic acid. The intermediate doses produced some epithelial scaling after about 4 or 5 days and was least with DBA and BP. It was most noticeable with DMBA when it was accompanied by some serous oozing in a few mice, mainly in areas that had been treated with acetic acid or croton oil. The largest doses of DBA and BP produced obvious keratin scaling but visible ulceration did not occur. The largest dose of DMBA (150 μg. per sq. cm.) produced severe changes in the skin submerging the effects of the preliminary treatments. There were often large areas of serous exudation which were slow in returning to normal, hair regrowth was delayed or in some cases did not occur, and the changes were accompanied by a constitutional disturbance.

The mice treated with the highest dose of DMBA did not gain as much in weight as those in the other groups. At the end of 30 weeks the animals were not in very good condition and, as the death rate appeared to be increasing, the experiments with DMBA were terminated at this time. Three of the mice treated with the highest dose of DMBA developed sarcomas associated with the thoracic cage and 4 of them developed a total of 6 papillomata well outside the treated area (which are not counted in the results). The occurrence of these tumours must be ascribed to absorption of the DMBA, which also may account for the deterioration in condition of these animals. In all the other groups the mice remained in better condition and the death rates were not so great. These experiments were continued for 40 weeks.

In the mice of Experiment III treated with 150 μg. per sq. cm. of DMBA and a preliminary application of acetic acid at the same time and 1 day beforehand, a crop of small papillary growths occurred on the skin from the 8th week, a total of 7 on the side treated with acetic acid and 2 on the untreated side; these lesions regressed rapidly and do not appear in the results. This crop of transient lesions was not seen in Experiment IV in the mice given the preliminary application of croton oil before DMBA.

The time of appearance of each tumour counted, the tumours that regressed and those that became malignant, on each mouse, are set out in Tables I to IV. The mice that died with tumours are also shown.

The statistical analysis for Experiments I, II and III is based on the actual counts of tumours at each 10-week interval recorded in Table II; and for Experiment IV on the actual count at the termination of the experiment, Table IV.

Experiments I, II and III

Although the mice in these 3 experiments were randomized, the tumour yields were too small to allow the data to be treated as a whole and the experiments were considered individually.

Experiment I—DBA.—The number of tumours was too small to estimate the effects of the various factors. At 40 weeks the total of 12 tumours on the right side treated with acetic acid, combining the results of the 3 dose levels, is significantly greater than the total of 3 tumours on the left untreated side ($\chi_1^2 = 5\cdot4$, $P < 0\cdot05$).

Experiment III—DMBA.—Firstly, it was noted that the number of tumours on the right side is significantly greater than on the left side, after 10 weeks, 20 weeks and 30 weeks for dose 150 μg. per sq. cm. and after 20 weeks and 30 weeks for dose 37 μg. per sq. cm.

The tumour yields were treated as Poisson type counts, and analysis of variance performed after the square root transformation was applied.

The analysis showed that the differences between the right side and the left side, for the dose 150 μg. per sq. cm., were not related to the number of weeks of observation ($F_{2\cdot6} = 0\cdot77$) but depended on the length of the interval between treatments ($F_{3\cdot6} = 22\cdot51$, $P < 0\cdot01$). For dose 37 μg. per sq. cm. the difference between right and left sides again depended on the interval between treatments ($F_{3\cdot3} = 92\cdot49$, $P < 0\cdot01$), but was not related to the period of observation ($F_{1\cdot3} = 7\cdot67$, $P > 0\cdot5$).

Experiment II—BP.—A similar analysis was made to that for DMBA using the 20-, 30- and 40-week data for dose level 150 μg. per sq. cm. but only the 30- and 40-week data for dose 37 μg. per sq. cm. At 40 weeks the total yield of 22 tumours, combining the results of all dose levels, on the right side is significantly greater than the 9 tumours on the left side. Analysis of variance of the right *versus* left side differences at the 150 μg. per sq. cm. dose level gave no significant effect for weeks of observation ($F_{2\cdot6} = 0\cdot87$) but a significant effect for interval between treatments ($F_{3\cdot6} = 17\cdot37$, $P < 0\cdot01$). For the 37 μg. per sq. cm. dose level neither effect is significant (for intervals between treatments $F_{3\cdot3} = 5\cdot20$, $P > 0\cdot1$), presumably because of the smallness of the yields.

Experiment IV

To consider the results of the individual carcinogens, in the mice treated with DMBA there are significant differences between the tumour yields ($\chi_4{}^2 = 14\cdot236$, $P < 0\cdot01$). The control group, given no preliminary treatment, differs significantly from the pretreated groups ($\chi_1{}^2 = 5\cdot074$, $P < 0\cdot05$) and there are significant differences between the pretreated groups ($\chi_3{}^2 = 9\cdot162$, $P < 0\cdot05$).

TABLE I.—*Influence of a Preliminary Application of Acetic Acid at Intervals before Application of Hydrocarbon on Distribution and Time of Appearance of Tumours*

Carcinogen	Dose. μg. per sq. cm.	Interval between treatments	Survivors at 20 weeks	Distribution and time of appearance of tumours on each mouse (Left side/Right side)
DBA	75	0	28	34/0; 0/*24*; 0/22; 0/28, (22); 0/30
		1	26	36/0; 0/26; 0/32
		3	27	32/0; 0/32
		9	25	0/(20); 0/34
	37	0	27	0/22
		1	23	(22)/0; 0/32
		3	23	No tumours.
		9	28	0/24
	9	0	30	0/28
		1	29	No tumours.
		3	25	0/(24); (28)/0
		9	30	No tumours.
BP	150	0	26	0/36; 34/28, *16*; 0/16, *18*; 24/*16*, 24; 0/32
		1	27	28/0; 34/*24*; 0/18, 30; 0/26; 0/36
		3	27	(26), 28/*16*, *18*; 0/30
		9	27	28/0; 0/(30)
	37	0	23	28/30; 0/28, 34
		1	28	24/0; 0/26, 24
		3	30	No tumours.
		9	28	36/0
	9	0	25	No tumours.
		1	27	0/26
		3	27	No tumours.
		9	27	No tumours.
DMBA	150	0	23*	20/(12), 22, 26; 0/22; 0/*12*; 0/*12*; 0/*12*, *16*, (12); [0/18]; 12/*12*; 0/*16*, 16, 18, 24; 0/(14); 0/22; 18/(22); 0/20, (18); 0/*14*, *16*, 24; [0/*16*, *16*]; [14/16, 18]
		1	22	0/22; 0/10, 14; (10)/(12), *12*, 14; 24/0; 24/(12); 0/10; 20/0; 22/(10); 0/(12), *16*; 0/22; [0/*16*, 22]
		3	22	22/0; 0/*16*, 19; 0/22, (12), (14); *12*, (14)/14; 0/22; 0/22, (10); 24/(22); 0/(18); 0/*16*
		9	28	(10)/0; 16/0; 14/10; 22/(10); [0/18]; *12*/0; (24)/0; 0/*12*
	37	0	25	0/14; 22/*12*, 18; 0/18; 0/16; 0/(16); 0/*12*; 22/0; 0/20, 22
		1	28	0/16; 0/18, 18, 18, 24; 0/24
		3	24	(16)/0
		9	26	0/24; 24/26; 22/0; 24/22, (24)
	9	0	28	0/22; 0/(18)
		1	28	0/*14*; 0/24
		3	28	No tumours.
		9	28	(12)/0; 22/(16)

Figures in parentheses are times of appearance of tumours that regressed.
Figures in italics are times of appearance of tumours that became malignant.
Figures in square brackets refer to mice that died with tumours.
* Tumours that appeared at ten weeks and regressed before twenty weeks are not shown.

TABLE II.—*The Influence of Preliminary Treatment with Acetic Acid on Number of Tumours Produced by Hydrocarbons*

Carcinogen	Interval between treatments	150 µg. per sq. cm. (BP and DMBA; DBA 75 µg. per sq. cm.) Surviving mice			37 µg. per sq. cm. Surviving mice			9 µg. per sq. cm. Surviving mice		
		Number of mice	Left side	Right side	Number of mice	Left side	Right side	Number of mice	Left side	Right side
DBA (40 weeks)	0	25	1	4	24	0	1	25	0	1
	1	24	1	2	22	0	1	28	0	1
	3	25	1	1	23	0	0	21	0	0
	9	22	0	1	24	0	1	27	0	0
DBA (30 weeks)	0	28	0	3	26	0	1	26	0	1
	1	26	0	1	22	0	0	28	1	0
	3	26	0	0	23	0	0	23	0	1
	9	23	0	1*	26	0	1	28	0	0
BP (40 weeks)	0	21	2	8	23	1	3	24	0	0
	1	23	2	5	26	1	2	26	0	1
	3	24	1	3	25	0	0	24	0	0
	9	25	1	0	27	1	0	23	0	0
BP (30 weeks)	0	21	1	6	23	1	2	24	0	0
	1	23	1	4	28	1	2	27	0	1
	3	25	2	3	30	0	0	27	0	0
	9	25	1	1	27	0	0	27	0	0
BP (20 weeks)	0	26	0	4	23	0	0	25	0	0
	1	27	0	1	28	0	0	27	0	0
	3	27	0	2	30	0	0	27	0	0
	9	27	0	0	28	0	0	27	0	0
DMBA (30 weeks)	0	19	3	17	24	2	8	25	0	1
	1	17	4	8	23	1	6	24	0	2
	3	16	3	7	24	0	0	28	0	0
	9	22	4	2	26	3	3	26	1	0
DMBA (20 weeks)	0	23	4	16	25	1	6	28	0	1
	1	22	1	10	28	0	4	28	0	1
	3	22	1	4	24	1	0	28	0	0
	9	28	4	3	26	0	0	28	1	1
DMBA (10 weeks)	0	23	2	22	27	0	0	30	0	0
	1	26	2	10	29	0	0	29	0	0
	3	28	4	9	26	0	0	29	0	0
	9	29	1	2	29	0	0	30	0	0

30 mice in each group at beginning of experiment.   * Present at 20 weeks.

75

TABLE III.—*Influence of a Preliminary Application of Croton Oil at Various Intervals before Application of Hydrocarbons on the Yield of Tumours and Times of Appearance of Tumours*

Carcinogen	Dose. µg. per sq. cm.	Interval between treatments	Survivors at 20 weeks	Distribution and time of appearance of tumours on each mouse (Right side/Left side)
DBA (40 weeks)	75	0	33	34/0; 28/*20*, (32); 34/0; 28/0; (32)/0; [0/20]
		1	34	34/0; 28/36, (34); 0/22
		3	32	36/0; 22/0; 0/28
		9	37	No tumours.
		A	36	36/0; (24)/0; 0/32
BP (40 weeks)	75	0	34	24/0; 22/18; 18, 22/22, 32, (24); 0/36; [(22)/*16*, 22]
		1	34	36/0; 24/18; 32/*18*, 24; 28/24, 28; (24)/36; 0/24, 34
		3	34	(20)/0; *18*, 32/28; 26/24, 32; 0/24
		9	35	22, 28, 36/0; 0/30; 0/32
		A	39	28/0; 32/36, (22)
DMBA (30 weeks)	75	0	29	*12*, 18/0; 18/(22), ·24; 24/0; 20/*14*, *18*, (18); (16), 22/16; 0/14; [0/*12*, 16]; [*10*, 18, 20/0]
		1	33	*12*, 16/18; *16*, *18*, (18), 24/12, 22; 16/20; 0/*18*, 22; 24/0; 16/*14*; 16, 24/20, 22; 18/0; 22, 26/0; [24/0]
		3	28	16, (18), (18)/20; 20, 22/0; 12/18, (22); 26/18, 24; 0/18, 22; 0/12, (20); (20)/24
		9	30	12/*10*; 22/0; 20/18, (18), (24), 24; (16)/16, 24
		A	34	12/0; 20/*14*, (18); 16/22; 24/0; (24)/(24)

Figures in parentheses are times of appearance of tumours that regressed.
Figures in italics are times of appearance of tumours that became malignant.
Figures in square brackets refer to mice that died with tumours.
Forty mice in each group at beginning of experiment.
Groups A had no preliminary treatment with croton oil.

TABLE IV.—*The Influence of Preliminary Treatment with Croton Oil on Number of Tumours Produced by Hydrocarbons*

	Interval between treatments	Surviving mice Number of mice	Surviving mice Mice with tumours	Surviving mice Number of tumours
DBA, 75 µg./sq. cm. (40 weeks)	0	29	4	5
	1	29	3	4
	3	28	3	3
	9	31	0	0
	A	32	2	2
BP, 75 µg./sq. cm. (40 weeks)	0	31	4	8
	1	29	6	12
	3	27	3	5
	9	30	3	5
	A	34	2	3
DMBA, 75 µg./sq. cm. (30 weeks)	0	25	6	11
	1	27	9	22
	3	26	7	13
	9	28	4	8
	A	30	4	6

Groups A had *no* preliminary treatment. Forty mice in each group at beginning of experiment.

In the mice treated with BP no very significant differences appear (overall $\chi_4^2 = 8\cdot428$, $P > 0\cdot05$; difference between control and pretreated groups $\chi_1^2 = 3\cdot409$, $P > 0\cdot05$; differences between pretreated groups $\chi_3^2 = 5\cdot019$, $P > 0\cdot10$). Similarly no significant differences appear in the mice treated with DBA.

For an analysis of variance, if it is assumed that the difference due to the intervals between treatments can be estimated independently of the carcinogen used, the data can be treated as a 3×5 factorial (3 carcinogens *versus* 4 pre-treatments and a control group). Tumour yields were treated as Poisson type counts.

Significant differences appear between the 3 carcinogens ($F_{2\cdot8} = 21\cdot43$, $P < 0\cdot001$). There are also significant differences between the control groups A and the pretreatment groups ($F_{1\cdot8} = 7\cdot414$, $P < 0\cdot05$). In addition, significant differences exist between the 4 pretreatment groups ($F_{3\cdot8} = 6\cdot489$, $P < 0\cdot05$). Comparing the pretreated groups with the controls the differences at the 0 interval and the 1 day interval are significant, $P < 0\cdot05$, and $P < 0\cdot01$ respectively. The difference between the controls and the 3 day interval is of doubtful significance and the remaining difference not significant at all.

In summary, there is clear evidence that, when one side of the skin of the back of mice is treated with acetic acid before application of any of the 3 hydrocarbons to the whole area of the skin of the back, the number of tumours produced is greater on the pretreated side. In the case of DMBA at the 150 μg. per sq. cm. and 37 μg. per sq. cm. dose levels and in the case of BP at the 150 μg. per sq. cm. dose level the increase varied with the interval between the 2 treatments and was independent of the period of observation. The tumour yields were increased when there was no significant interval between the 2 treatments and at an interval of 24 hours. A similar trend appears at the lower dose levels of DMBA and BP and also when DBA was the carcinogen although the tumour yields were too small for statistical treatment.

Similarly when mice were given a preliminary treatment with croton oil before the application of the carcinogens the tumour yield was increased when the interval between treatments was zero and 24 hours. A doubtful effect was found at an interval of 3 days. The variation with the interval between treatments is significant only with DMBA, but a similar trend is seen in the results with DBA and BP.

From inspection of Tables I and III it is apparent that these trends are maintained in mice that died with tumours. Also, the number of tumours that regressed was greater on skin that had the preliminary treatment.

It is to be noted that the tumour yields in areas of skin that did not have the preliminary treatment with acetic acid (in Experiments I, II, and III), appear to be similar, allowing for variation in dosage levels, to the tumour yields in mice that had no pretreatment with croton oil in Experiment IV. Similarly, in areas of skin subjected to preliminary treatment with acetic acid in Experiments I, II and III the increase in tumour yields is of similar order to the increase in the tumour yields in similar areas of mice that had a preliminary treatment with croton oil, again allowing for the variation in dosage levels.

It will be observed from Tables I and III that tumours appear earlier on the average with the more potent carcinogens. The tumour yields are not such as to treat this statistically.

Lastly, it is apparent from Tables I and III that malignant tumours appear to be more frequent in areas given the preliminary treatment on the one hand and with the more potent carcinogens on the other. However, the ratio of malignant to benign tumours does not vary significantly between the different areas. The frequency of malignant tumours therefore appears to be related to the number of tumours in any particular area, and perhaps also to the length of time tumours have been under observation.

DISCUSSION

The production of skin tumours in mice by a single application of a carcinogenic hydrocarbon has been reported, for example, using 3 : 4-benzopyrene (Biels-chowsky and Bullough, 1949), 20-methylcholanthrene (Mider and Morton, 1939; Cramer and Stowell, 1943) and 9 : 10-dimethyl-1 : 2-benzanthracene (Law, 1941; Andreasen and Engelbreth-Holm, 1953; Borum, 1954; Terracini, Shubik and Porta, 1960). The tumours appeared in small numbers after a long latent period; most have been benign but some were malignant. Allowing for the differing strains of mice used by different workers and for the uncertainties of dosage per unit area of skin, DMBA appears to be the most active as judged by the numbers of tumours produced.

The number of tumours to be expected in the experiments reported in this paper is therefore likely to be small, as was found, although a quantitative comparison of the results with those of other authors is invalid because of the differing strains of mice, uncertainty in the dosage per unit area used by other authors, the particular sample of DMBA, DBA and BP used and possibly other factors. Dose-response data have been reported with DMBA (Terracini et al., 1960) and the present results follow a similar pattern. Nonetheless, it is clear that DMBA produced more tumours than DBA or BP, and that BP was more active than DBA, at least with the samples used.

A preliminary application of acetic acid or croton oil at the same time as, or a short interval before, the application of any of the 3 hydrocarbons increased the number of tumours produced. The relative increase when the treated side of mice that had the preliminary treatment of acetic acid on one side of the skin of the back was compared with the untreated side was similar to the relative increase when mice that had a preliminary treatment with croton oil to the whole of the back were compared with mice that had no preliminary treatment. The augmenting effect is therefore localized to the area affected by the preliminary treatment and not the result of general metabolic changes; although formal demonstration of this would depend on the results of similar experiments in which the manner of the preliminary treatments were reversed. However, since the tumour yields in untreated areas of skin in the 2 experiments were similar, these experiments would appear to be redundant. The amounts of acetic acid or croton oil applied were the highest that could be used without producing clinical ulceration of the skin and led to similar degrees of epithelial scaling as judged by the naked eye.

Croton oil is a potent promoting agent for the production of skin tumours in mice subjected to the action of an initiating agent such as urethane (Salaman and Roe, 1953) or the carcinogenic hydrocarbons (Mottram, 1944a; Berenblum and Shubik, 1947); and on repeated application alone appears to have a minor carcino-genic effect (Roe, 1956; Boutwell, Bosch and Rusch, 1957). However, acetic acid has no promoting activity when carcinogenic hydrocarbons are employed as initiating agents and does not itself lead to the production of tumours (Gwynn and Salaman, 1953). The tumour augmenting effect is therefore, as in the case of the similar augmenting effect of preliminary irritation on urethane carcinogenesis (Pound and Withers, 1963; Pound, 1966), not related to these properties but is probably related to the common property of producing inflammation and cell proliferation in the skin.

However, in the case of experiments in which hydrocarbons are applied to the skin, other factors merit consideration. Thus, the number of tumours produced after a single application of DMBA appears to be related to the stage of the hair cycle at the time, more tumours being produced if this is in the resting phase (Andreasen and Engelbreth-Holm, 1953; Borum, 1954). From study of sections of mice of the same age and weight, the hair cycle of about one-third the mice used in the present experiments is in the late catagen phase and of the remainder in the resting phase. The possibility that the results can be due to a variation from this source is therefore unlikely and can be excluded since treated sides were compared with the untreated sides of the same animals in which the cycle would be in the same phase on either side. However, it has been shown that the hair cycle effect is explained mainly by retention of the hydrocarbon in the resting hair follicles (Berenblum, Haran-Ghera and Trainin, 1958).

After the application of croton oil in the amount used, vascular dilatation and oedema develop rapidly and increase to about the 12th hour, after which the changes regress slowly to approach normal after about 24 hours. These changes are accompanied by a leucocytic infiltration which, however, persists for longer than 24 hours. The number of nuclei of the epidermis labelled in radio-autographs of sections of the skin, when the mice were injected with 10 μc tritiated thymidine 30 minutes before being killed, increased very rapidly from the 9th hour to a maximum at the 18th hour and then receded to normal at about the 9th day, whereas mitotic counts in the epidermis increased slowly from the 15th hour to a maximum at about 36 hours and then receded slowly to normal at about the 9th day (Pound, 1968). A similar pattern of these events was reported by Iversen and Evensen (1962). Forty-eight hours after the application of croton oil the epidermis is increased in thickness and soon begins to differentiate a layer of keratin. The epidermal changes extend into the superficial part of the hair follicles. Although no study has been made of the changes following an application of acetic acid, the changes visible to the naked eye are similar and the microscopic events are likely to be substantially the same.

It seems possible that the proliferating epidermis, on the surface and in the superficial part of the hair follicles, might have an increased capacity to retain hydrocarbons applied to the skin but if this factor contributed significantly to the results, the tumour yield would be expected to be augmented when the hydrocarbon was applied on the 3rd and 9th days after the preliminary application. This was not the case.

In previous studies concerning the augmenting effect of irritants on tumour initiation by urethane (Pound, 1968) it has been shown that the increased tumour yield correlates with cellular events in the skin, in particular with the number of cells replicating DNA, at the time of injection of the urethane. This suggests that this chemical exerts its tumour initiating action during this phase.

It seems possible that the carcinogenic hydrocarbons also act during a similar period of the cell cycle. The demonstration of this in experiments in which the hydrocarbon is applied to the skin is likely to be clouded by the facts that, on the one hand, these compounds persist in the tissue for a considerable time, and, on the other hand, they themselves lead to epithelial hyperplasia in the skin (Orr, 1938). The sharp increase in tumour yields found when urethane was injected as an initiating agent at various times after a preliminary irritating treatment of the skin could not be expected. This indeed was the reason for selection of the particular intervals between the preliminary treatment and the application of the hydrocarbon used in the present experiments.

Many years ago Mottram (1944*b*) reported that the number of tumours produced by benzopyrene (used as an initiating agent followed by repeated applications of cróton oil which he referred to as a developing factor, but which is now referred to as a promoting agent) was increased if the skin was given a preliminary treatment with croton oil. He showed that the preliminary treatment resulted in a great increase in the mitotic counts in the skin. Similarly, he found that a preliminary treatment with cantharidin under conditions that depressed the mitotic counts decreased the tumour yields, and under conditions that increased the mitotic counts cantharidin increased the tumour yields. Mottram (1945) also found that more tumours were produced if the benzopyrene was applied at midnight rather than at midday which he ascribed to higher mitotic rates at this time, a view that has not been supported by subsequent results (Bielschowsky and Bullough, 1949). He concluded that "the genesis of tumours represents action on cell division". In spite of the revolutionary nature of this concept, for various reasons experiments that would confirm or refute this thesis have only been performed recently.

Frei and Ritchie (1964) have confirmed that DMBA, followed by promoting treatment with croton oil, produces more tumours if applied at midnight than if applied at midday; and Shinozuka and Ritchie (1967) have reported that a preliminary application of croton oil 23 hours before the application of DMBA, as an initiating agent, augmented the yield of tumours. These results were interpreted as compatible with the theory that the carcinogens act on cells synthesizing DNA.

A similar result was reported (Pound, 1968) using DBA as an initiating agent but the tumour yield was increased at intervals of 0, 24 hours and 3 days, and not at 9 days, between a preliminary application of acetic acid and the carcinogen. Almost identical results have been obtained (Pound, to be published) when BP and DMBA were the initiating agents. While these results completely dissociate the augmenting effect of the preliminary treatment from promoting activity, they do not give the clear correlation with the pattern of DNA synthesis found with urethane. Nor should such a pattern be expected for reasons noted above. In further experiments (Pound, 1968) it was reported that partial hepatectomy before injection of urethane or oral administration of DMBA increased the number of tumours produced in the liver, an effect that may be related to the active regeneration of the liver during the presence of the carcinogen.

It seems possible therefore that tissues induced to proliferate rapidly become more susceptible to the action of a carcinogen, as a general phenomenon. The evidence that possibly identifies the sensitive phase in cell life as the phase of replication of DNA comes mainly from the work with urethane (Pound, 1968).

The author thanks Dr. H. Silverstone, Reader in Medical Statistics, for the statistical analysis. This work was partly supported by a grant from the Queensland Cancer Fund.

REFERENCES

ANDREASEN, E., AND ENGELBRETH-HOLM, J.—(1953) Acta path. microbiol. scand., 32, 165.
BERENBLUM, I., HARAN-GHERA, NECHAMA, AND TRAININ, N.—(1958) Br. J. Cancer, 12, 402.
BERENBLUM, I., AND SHUBIK, P.—(1947) Br. J. Cancer, 1, 379.
BIELSCHOWSKY, F. AND BULLOUGH, W. S.—(1949) Br. J. Cancer, 3, 282.
BORUM, K.—(1954) Acta path. microbiol. scand., 34, 542.
BOUTWELL, R. K., BOSCH, D. AND RUSCH, H. P.—(1957) Cancer Res., 17, 71.
CRAMER, W. AND STOWELL, R. E.—(1943) Cancer Res., 3, 36.
FREI, J. V. AND RITCHIE, A. C.—(1964) J. natn. Cancer Inst., 32, 1213.
GWYNN, R. H. AND SALAMAN, M. H.—(1953) Br. J. Cancer, 7, 482.
IVERSEN, O. H. AND EVENSEN, A.—(1962) Acta path. microbiol. scand. Supp. 156.
LAW, L. W.—(1941) Am. J. Path., 17, 827.
MIDER, G. B. AND MORTON, J. J.—(1939) Am. J. Path., 15, 299.
MOTTRAM, J. C.—(1944a) J. Path. Bact., 56, 181.—(1944b) J. Path. Bact., 56, 391.
MOTTRAM, J. C.—(1945) J. Path. Bact., 57, 265.
ORR, J. W.—(1938) J. Path. Bact., 46, 495.
POUND, A. W.—(1962) Br. J. Cancer, 16, 246.
POUND, A. W.—(1963) Aust. J. exp. Biol. med. Sci., 41, 73.
POUND, A. W.—(1966) Br. J. Cancer, 20, 385.
POUND, A. W.—(1968) Proceedings of the First New Zealand International Symposium on Cancer, University of Otago, Dunedin, November, 1966. N.Z. med. J. (Special Issue), 67, 88.
POUND, A. W. AND WITHERS, H. R.—(1963) Br. J. Cancer, 17, 460.
ROE, F. J. C.—(1956) Br. J. Cancer, 10, 72.
SALAMAN, M. H. AND ROE, F. J. C.—(1953) Br. J. Cancer, 7, 472.
SHINOZUKA, H. AND RITCHIE, A. C.—(1967) Int. J. Cancer, 2, 77.
TERRACINI, B., SHUBIK, P. AND PORTA, G. D.—(1960) Cancer Res.. 20. 1538.

Tumor Promotion by 1-Fluoro-2,4-dinitrobenzene, a Potent Skin Sensitizer[1]

Fred G. Bock, Audrey Fjelde, Helen W. Fox, and Edmund Klein

INTRODUCTION

In recent years, growing attention has been given to the relationship between chemical carcinogens and the immunologic system in experimental animals. Stjernsward (11, 12) reported an immunodepressive effect of polycyclic hydrocarbons which reduced reaction against weak antigenic homografts. Rubin (10) showed that in certain situations intensive treatment of mice with carcinogenic benz[α]anthracene derivatives abolished the rejection of tumors that differ from the host, even at the strongly antigenic H-2 locus. He suggested that this involved "an active immunologic process initiated by carcinogen treatment." Other skin carcinogens with different molecular structures had the same effect (5). Prehn (8) provided a scheme by which positive selection favoring immunologically different malignant cell lines, together with suppression of the immune response of the host, might account for chemical carcinogenesis.

A similarity in the immunologic properties of polycyclic carcinogens, croton oil, and 1-fluoro-2,4-dinitrobenzene (DNFB) was recently reported by Fjelde and Turk (4). It had been shown that topical application of DNFB to the skin of guinea pigs was followed by the appearance of large pyroninophilic cells in draining lymph nodes 4 days later, one day before the animals developed contact sensitivity (13). Fjelde and Turk obtained a similar result when guinea pigs or any of 5 strains

[1]This study was supported in part by Grant E386 from the American Cancer Society.

of mice were treated with either of the potent carcinogens benzo[α]pyrene and 7,12-dimethylbenz[α]anthracene (DMBA). Croton oil, which is primarily a tumor promoter (3), produced a similar result in the single strain of mice tested. In contrast, the noncarcinogenic hydrocarbon anthracene was inactive in both mice and guinea pigs.

This similarity among the complete carcinogens, the tumor promoter croton oil, and the immunologically active DNFB, together with the observed effects of carcinogens in homograft rejection, led us to determine whether DNFB might act as a carcinogen or tumor promoter in the mouse skin system. In an earlier study, Fjelde et al.[2] obtained no tumors when DNFB was applied in croton oil to mice under conditions providing severe immunologic response. DNFB thus did not seem to be an effective tumor initiator. The present report describes the tumor-promoting activity of this interesting compound.

MATERIALS AND METHODS

DMBA and DNFB were obtained from Distillation Products Industries, Rochester, N. Y. N^6-(2,4-Dinitrophenyl)-L-lysine hydrochloride (DNPL) was obtained from Mann Research Laboratories, New York, N. Y. All compounds were used without further purification. The concentration of the DMBA solutions used in the study was checked with a spectrophotometer. Solutions of DNFB and DNPL in acetone were prepared fresh daily.

To test DNFB as a tumor-initiating agent, 60 female ICR Swiss mice were treated at 55 and 62 days of age with 0.25 ml of a 1% solution of DNFB in a 1:1 mixture of acetone and sesame oil. Of the 60 mice, 22 died following the second treatment. After 7 days, the remaining 38 mice were treated 5 times a week for 30 weeks with 0.25 ml of 0.03% croton oil in acetone. A group of 30 mice, treated with the croton oil solution alone, served as negative controls.

To determine whether DNFB was a promoting agent, groups of 30 female ICR Swiss mice were painted at 55 days of age with 125 μg of DMBA in 0.25 ml of acetone. After 21 days, the mice were treated 5 times a week with 0.25 ml of acetone

---

[2]A. Fjelde, E. Sorkin, and T. Strauli. Immunological Factors and Tumor Development. I. Studies of Leukocytes from Fluoro-2,4-dinitrobenzene Treated Mice Challenged in Tissue Culture with Dinitrophenyl-lysine. Submitted for publication.

solutions of DNFB ranging in concentration from 0.03% to 3%. One group of 30 mice, treated with DMBA followed by acetone, served as negative controls; another group, treated with DMBA followed by paintings 5 times a week with 0.03% croton oil in acetone, served as positive controls. The experiment was continued for 32 weeks, after which the animals were used for other studies (7).

A second experiment was designed to repeat the first, and to determine whether DNFB might have acted through nonspecific conjugates formed with amino acids, peptides, or proteins. Groups of 50 female ICR Swiss mice were treated with DMBA as before. After 3 weeks, one group was treated with 0.1% DNFB in 0.25 ml of acetone 5 times a week. A second group was treated with 0.5% of DNPL, the lysine conjugate of DNFB, in a 3:1 mixture of acetone and water 5 times a week. The third group consisted of 50 mice that were not treated with DMBA but were treated only with 0.1% DNFB 5 times a week throughout the experiment. Two control groups consisted of mice treated with DMBA followed by either acetone or 0.03% croton oil in acetone as before. A second series consisted of groups of 30 C57BL/6 mice, 15 of each sex, which were treated with DMBA followed by acetone, croton oil, or 0.1% DNFB as in the other studies. A third experiment involved 12 male and 18 female BALB/c mice treated with DMBA followed by acetone, 0.03% croton oil, or 0.1% DNFB.

The mice were examined at weekly intervals, and the distribution of skin tumors was noted. In all, the three experiments covered a time span of 13 months.

The apparent toxic effects of DNFB were more pronounced in the mice treated with DMBA. To determine whether this observation was real, 7 groups of mice were painted with various combinations of DMBA and DNFB (Table 1). The schedule was arranged so that, for each group, the DNFB treatment commenced on the same day and followed the last DMBA treatment by 7 days. To provide objective evidence of toxicity, a 0.2% as well as a 0.1% solution of DNFB was employed.

RESULTS

DNFB proved to be quite toxic under the experimental conditions. Animals painted with either a 3% or a 1% solution of this compound in acetone died after a single application. Of 30 mice, 6 died after 8 applications of 0.3% DNFB in acetone. The Swiss and C57BL/6 mice treated with either 0.1% or 0.03% DNFB in acetone appeared to tolerate the compound, but the BALB/c mice were more sensitive. The experiment with BALB/c mice was terminated after 14 weeks with only 14 mice surviving out of the original 30. Indications that com-

84

Table 1

Group	DMBA (μg)	DNFB[a] (%)	Total no. of mice	No. dead
1	3 X 125[b]	0.1	10	1
2	125[c]	0.1	10	1
3	0	0.1	10	0
4	125[c]	0.2	10	6
5	0	0.2	10	0
6	125[c]	0	8	0
7	0	0	8	0

Potentiation of acute 1-fluoro-2,4-dinitrobenzene (DNFB) toxicity by 7,12-dimethylbenz[α]anthracene (DMBA).

[a]0.25 ml of acetone solution applied 5 times a week for 4 weeks beginning at 82 days of age.

[b]0.25 ml of acetone solution applied at 61, 68, and 75 days of age.

[c]0.25 ml of acetone solution applied at 75 days of age.

bined treatment with DMBA plus DNFB was more toxic than DNFB alone were confirmed. The lethal effects of 0.2% DNFB were significantly greater when the mice were first treated with DMBA (Table 1).

DNFB also proved to be a very potent tumor-promoting agent (Table 2). Indeed, the first tumors produced by this agent appeared after 4 weeks of painting, whereas the first tumors produced by croton oil were seen only after 6 weeks. In each of the four experimental series, the first tumors appeared in the DNFB-treated mice. On the other hand, many more tumors were finally produced by croton oil treatment. Of 80 ICR Swiss mice treated with DMBA and 0.1% DNFB for 32 weeks, 51 developed papillomas. In the same time, 59 of 80 mice treated with DMBA and 0.03% croton oil developed tumors. The number of tumors per tumor-bearing mouse, however, was 5.7 with croton oil, but only 1.5 with DNFB. This difference in effects was less marked in the C57BL/6 mice (Table 3).

Although 0.1% DNFB was very toxic to the BALB/c mice, they developed tumors rapidly. Of 20 mice that survived 6 weeks, 5 had tumors by that time. The C57BL/6 mice developed fewer tumors than either the Swiss or the BALB/c mice;

Table 2

Initiating stimulus	Promoting stimulus[a]	No. of mice at risk[b]	Mice with tumors		Total no. of tumors	No. of mice in which tumors regressed
			No.	%		
None	0.03% croton oil	56	1	2	1	1
2 × 2500 μg DNFB	0.03% croton oil	38[d]	1	3	1	1
125 μg DMBA	None	30	0	0	0	0
	0.03% croton oil	30	15	50	79	0
	0.3% DNFB[c]	24	6	25	8	2
	0.1% DNFB	30	21	70	41	1
	0.03% DNFB	21	9	38	11	0

Tumor promotion by 1-fluoro-2,4-dinitrobenzene (DNFB).

[a] 0.25 ml of acetone solution 5 times a week for 32 weeks.
[b] ICR Swiss mice surviving at least 2 weeks of promoting stimulus.
[c] 6 of 30 mice died after only 8 applications of 0.3% DNFB; further treatment was discontinued.
[d] 22 of 60 mice died after the second DNFB treatment.

the first tumors appeared in the C57BL/6 mice after 10 weeks. The C57BL/6 mice were also less sensitive to croton oil.

The effect of DNFB showed a clear dose-response pattern. After only 8 applications, 0.3% DNFB produced tumors in 6 of 24 surviving animals. Although the final number of tumors produced by 0.03% DNFB was more than a third of that produced by 0.1% DNFB, most of the tumors produced by the dilute solution appeared very late in the experiment. After 26 weeks, only two tumors appeared in 2 mice painted with the dilute 0.03% solution, whereas 31 tumors appeared in 21 mice painted with 0.1% solution for 26 weeks.

A single tumor appeared in mice treated 2 times with 1% DNFB followed by croton oil for 32 weeks. A tumor also appeared in the croton oil controls. Thus, in this experiment, DNFB was not a tumor initiator. Furthermore, treatment with DNFB alone produced no tumors.

The lysine conjugate of DNFB produced no tumors in DMBA-treated mice even when applied at 0.5% (14 mM) concentration. In contrast, 0.03% DNFB (1.6 mM) produced tumors in 38% of DMBA-treated mice.

DISCUSSION

DNFB acted as a tumor promoter in the three stocks of mice that were studied. The compound did not demonstrate tumor-initiating activity when mice were painted twice with this material followed by repetitive application of croton oil. Likewise, treatment with DNFB alone did not produce tumors, as would be expected with a potent tumor promoter that also exhibited initiating activity. Failure to find initiating activity is in agreement with the earlier observation by Fjelde et al.[2] that DNFB dissolved in croton oil did not produce tumors in Rudiger mice.

None of the tumors promoted by DNFB grew to a large size during the experimental period. In this respect, the agent appears much more like croton oil than like the carcinogenic polycyclic hydrocarbons, which, if applied in doses producing tumors in 4 weeks, would produce a large number of malignant tumors well within a 30-week period. On the other hand, a comparison of the total numbers of tumors that developed shows a striking difference between croton oil and DNFB treatment. Although tumors appeared earlier with DNFB, many more tumors finally appeared after croton oil treatment.

To some extent, DNFB resembles anthralin, which is a very potent tumor promoter (2, 3). In an earlier study, 50% of 30 Swiss mice treated with 125 μg of DMBA followed by 0.033% anthralin in acetone developed tumors in 32 weeks (1). In the present study, 38% of 21 mice treated with 0.03% DNFB de-

Table 3

Strain of mouse	Promoting stimulus[a]	Duration of promotion (weeks)	No. of mice at risk	Mice with tumors		Total no. of tumors	Tumors per tumor-bearing mouse
				No.	%		
Swiss	0.1% DNFB[b]	50	50	35	70	55	1.6
C57BL/6		50	30	6	20	8	1.3
BALB/c		14	30	5	17	7	1.4
Swiss	Acetone only	50	50	2	4	2	1.0
C57BL/6		50	30	0	0	0	
BALB/c		14	30	0	0	0	
Swiss	0.03% croton oil	50	50	49	98	346	7.1
C57BL/6		50	30	20	67	35	1.8
BALB/c		14	30	5	17	8	1.6
Swiss	0.5% dinitrophenyllysine hydrochloride	34	50	0	0	0	

Tumor promotion by 1-fluoro-2,4-dinitrobenzene (DNFB) in various stocks of mice.
[a] 0.25 ml of acetone solutions, applied 5 times a week beginning 21 days after a single application of 125 μg of DMBA in 0.25 ml of acetone.
[b] 50 Swiss mice treated with 0.1% DNFB, but not with DMBA, developed no tumors in 38 weeks.

veloped tumors in the same period. Aside from the phorbol esters, the active agents of croton oil (6, 14), DNFB is one of the most potent tumor-promoting agents available.

DNFB may owe its tumor-promoting activity to direct chem-

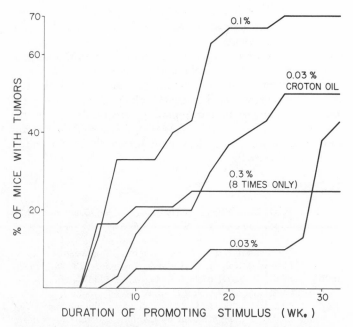

Chart 1. Dose-time response of tumor induction by 1-fluoro-2,4-dinitrobenzene (DNFB). Note in Table 2 that more tumors were induced by 0.03% croton oil than by 0.1% DNFB in spite of the fact that DNFB produced tumors earlier and in more mice than did croton oil. Mice bearing multiple tumors were rare in groups painted throughout the study with 0.03% DNFB or with 0.3% DNFB for eight applications only.

89

ical reaction with a specific active site. Conversely, its activity may be due to formation of a nonspecific conjugate with amino acids, peptides, or proteins, the conjugate being more directly involved in the expression of activity. The lysine conjugate of DNFB, N^6-(2,4-dinitrophenyl)-L-lysine, is immunologically active in some systems (4). In the present experiments, the lysine conjugate was inactive. This inactivity, however, does not preclude consideration of such conjugates as proximal promoting agents. The conjugate has substantially different solubility properties and might be inactive after skin application because of nonpenetration into the target areas. Lipid solubility is of great importance in skin penetration (1).

In these experiments, the DNFB was applied to the same site as the DMBA, and the tumors arose in the treated area. It might be considered whether the DNFB could exhibit systemic effects and promote tumors in initiated cells remote from the site of DNFB application. This would be the case if the progression from initiated cell to gross tumor depended on generalized sensitization to DNFB. Studies of this possibility are currently underway.

DNFB and 1-chloro-2,4-dinitrobenzene are well-known causes of allergic dermatitis. Many skin carcinogens of diverse structure alter the immune mechanisms of mice (4, 9—11; Footnote 2). Presumably they serve as both initiators and promoters. For several polycyclic hydrocarbons, initiating action can be distinguished from promoting action (8, 15). It is interesting to speculate that alterations in the immune system are a necessary feature of tumor-promoting activity. Two active tumor promoters, croton oil and DNFB, do mobilize pyroninophilic cells, a process which is immunologically specific in the latter case at least.

REFERENCES

1. Bock, F. G. Early Effects of Hydrocarbons on Mammalian Skin. Progr. Exptl. Tumor Res., 4: 126—168, 1964.

2. Bock, F. G., and Burns, R. Tumor-Promoting Properties of Anthralin (1,8,9-Anthratriol). J. Natl. Cancer Inst., 30: 393—398, 1963.
3. Boutwell, R. K. Some Biological Aspects of Skin Carcinogenesis. Progr. Exptl. Tumor Res., 4: 207—250, 1964.
4. Fjelde, A., and Turk, J. L. Induction of an Immunological Response in Local Lymph Nodes by Chemical Carcinogens. Nature, 205: 813—815, 1965.
5. Fox, H., and Bock, F. G. Chemical Specificity of Carcinogen-Induced Tolerance to Homotransplantation. J. Natl. Cancer Inst., 38: 789—795, 1967.
6. Hecker, E. Phorbol Esters from Croton Oil. Chemical Nature and Biological Activities. Naturwissenschaften, 54: 282—284, 1967.
7. Klein, E., MacEvoy, B., Milgrom, H., and Helm, F. Transfer of Cell

Mediated Immune Reactivity of Cutaneous Neoplasms. Proc. Am. Assoc. Cancer Res., *9:* 38, 1968.

8. Prehn, R. T. A Clonal Selection Theory of Chemical Carcinogenesis. J. Natl. Cancer Inst., *32:* 1–17, 1964.

9. Roe, F. J. C., and Salaman, M. H. Further Studies on Incomplete Carcinogenesis: Triethylene Melamine (T.E.M.), 1,2-Benzanthracene and β-Propiolactone as Initiators of Skin Tumour Formation in the Mouse. Brit. J. Cancer, *9:* 177–203, 1955.

10. Rubin, B. A. Carcinogen-Induced Tolerance to Homotransplantation. Progr. Exptl. Tumor Res., *5:* 217–292, 1964.

11. Stjernswärd, J. Immunodepressive Effect of 3-Methylcholanthrene. Antibody Formation at the Cellular Level and Reaction Against Weak Antigenic Homografts. J. Natl. Cancer Inst., *35:* 885–892, 1965.

12. Stjernswärd, J. Further Immunological Studies of Chemical Carcinogenesis. J. Natl. Cancer Inst., *38:* 515–526, 1967.

13. Turk, J. L., and Stone, S. H. Implications of the Cellular Changes in Lymph Nodes during the Development and Inhibition of Delayed Type Hypersensitivity. *In:* B. Amos and H. Koprowski (eds.), Cell-Bound Antibodies, pp. 51–60. Philadelphia: The Wistar Institute Press, 1963.

14. Van Duuren, B. L., and Orris, L. The Tumor-Enhancing Principles of *Croton tiglium L.* Cancer Res., *25:* 1871–1875, 1965.

15. Van Duuren, B. L., Sivak, A., Langseth, L., Goldschmidt, B. M., and Segal, A. Initiators and Promoters in Tobacco Carcinogenesis. Natl. Cancer Inst. Monogr., *28:* 173–180, 1968.

91

The Nature of Tumor-promoting Agents in Tobacco Products

Fred G. Bock

SUMMARY

The results available so far suggest to us the following tentative conclusions. First, there are at least two agents extracted by aqueous barium hydroxide from commercial cigarette tobacco that are required simultaneously in order to exhibit tumor-promoting activity. One of the agents is soluble in 80% methanol and is probably soluble in 95% methanol. The other is insoluble in 80% methanol and may consist of a single compound of molecular weight approximately 1600 or else consists of a spectrum of compounds, some of large molecular weight and some of molecular weight 1600 or smaller. The fraction of large molecular weight is the more active on a per gram basis. Second, the activity of aqueous extracts is higher with commercial cigarette preparations than with fresh tobacco leaf that has not been sprayed with chemical agents. We cannot determine whether this increase is due to an increase in one or the other of the two components or whether both are increased concurrently during cigarette manufacture. Furthermore, we do not yet know whether the increase occurs during the curing and aging of the leaf, whether it occurs during cigarette formulation, or whether it is due to particular cultural practices in growing the leaf.

In addition to those extracted with aqueous agents, other tumor promoters are extracted from tobacco with nonpolar solvents. It thus appears that the tumor-promoting activity of unburned tobacco products is due to various chemical compounds of highly different characteristics. Whether any of these play a role in the development of oral carcinoma is yet to be determined.

The tumor-promoting activity of cigarette smoke condensate cannot yet be related to the activity of the aqueous extracts of unburned tobacco. The promoting agents thus far demonstrated in cigarette smoke condensate are either phenolic or nonpolar in nature. No clear relationship between the aqueous extracts of unburned tobacco and cigarette smoke promoters is apparent.

INTRODUCTION

The role of tobacco products in the causation of malignant disease in man and in laboratory animals is well established (15, 16, 19). In man, tobacco products cause cancer in tissues directly exposed to them and, in addition, may be involved in the production of tumors in remote organs through metabolic change. Contact carcinogenesis induced by tobacco products is by far the most pronounced and thus the most thoroughly studied of these two modalities.

Tobacco products are relatively weak carcinogenic stimuli and are a health problem only because their intensive use is so widespread. But the weakness of their carcinogenicity, in combination with the chemical complexity of natural products, has made the evaluation of the tobacco carcinogens extraordinarily difficult. Although some clues to their nature may be obtained through epidemiologic studies, no clear-cut identification of these agents seems likely without recourse to laboratory investigation.

It has been possible to demonstrate a large number of carcinogens in tobacco products through conventional analytical methods. Nevertheless, there is no means of determining whether these carcinogens, at the concentrations involved, account for the tumors associated with the use of tobacco by human beings. Indeed, one of the most embarrassing problems to workers in this field is the fact that it has not yet been possible to identify the agents responsible for the carcinogenic activity exhibited by crude preparations of tobacco applied to the laboratory mouse.

Extracts of unburned cigarette tobacco as well as cigarette smoke condensate can serve as tumor-promoting agents (2, 17). That being the case, it is important to know whether the tumor promoters in unburned tobacco find their way into the smoke either in the original form or in an altered form that still retains the critically active functional groups. The evidence to be presented here suggests that at least some of the promoters in unburned tobacco are distinctly different from those in cigarette smoke.

Tumor Promoters in Cigarette Smoke Condensate. It has been suggested that, in man, cigarette smoke acts as a tumor promoter (6). In support of this hypothesis, a number of workers have shown that certain fractions of smoke condensate, and in particular the phenolic fraction, can act as tumor promoters (11, 18). Up to the present time, however, comparison of the promoting activity of any fraction with that of the crude condensate at corresponding dose levels has not been reported. One problem is that fractions that exhibit complete

93

carcinogenic activity would also exhibit promoting activity. It now appears that the bulk of the promoting activity of smoke condensate is accounted for by the phenolic fraction and various subfractions of the neutral fraction. Ether-soluble bases are of marginal activity.

Tumor Promoters in Unburned Tobacco. There is substantial literature describing the association of betel chewing with oral carcinoma (13). Most authors, but not all (1), attribute a large part of the oral carcinoma of the Far East to the use of tobacco in the betel quid. In the United States, the chewing of snuff is associated with both oral carcinoma and leukoplakia (7, 12). In many cases, it has been established that the tumor appears at the site where the quid is held. It is conceivable that the lesions are due solely to continuous trauma, but it seems more reasonable to entertain a hypothesis that chemical constituents of the quid are also involved. Davis (5), Orr (9), and Chang (4) have suggested that the use of lime in the betel quid adds to the potency of the preparation. Lime could act through its caustic effects on the tissues or through alkaline degradation of complex plant constituents into active smaller molecules.

To look for carcinogens in unburned tobacco, we therefore employed two extracts, one using organic solvents and the other using aqueous barium hydroxide as the extracting solution. In the latter case, the barium ion was removed effectively by carbon dioxide so that the final solution would not be caustic. The extracts were tested by application to the shaved backs of ICR Swiss mice after a single prior treatment with 125 μg of 7,12-dimethylbenz[α]anthracene (DMBA) in 0.25 ml of acetone. In this study and in all of those to follow, 0.25 ml of the extract was applied 5 times weekly throughout the experiment, which was usually terminated after 26 weeks. Both the acetone extract and the aqueous barium hydroxide extract contained tumor-promoting agents (2). Neither fraction exhibited significant complete carcinogenic activity; but the extracts were studied near the lower limit of detection, and complete carcinogenic stimuli would not have been detected in such concentrations. It was not possible to make quantitative comparison between the acetone and aqueous solutions, but it seemed to us that more activity per cigarette was demonstrated by the aqueous extract. It was likewise impossible to determine whether the two extracts contained the same or completely different agents. We chose to investigate the aqueous extract further.

Characteristics of the Water-soluble Promoters. The design of the biologic assays was such that the effects of experimental manipulation on the tumor-promoting agents could be determined. In every experiment involving fractionation, a recon-

94

stituted product was obtained by blending the various fractions in proportion to the yield obtained. Thus, if there was no effect of experimental manipulation, the reconstituted fraction was identical in all respects with the starting material. For ease of comparison, the dose employed is reported on the basis of cigarette equivalents per week (CEW), i.e., the number of cigarettes extracted to obtain the weekly dose used per mouse. The crude extracts employed to provide 2.5 CEW contained 0.6 to 0.8 gm of solids per milliliter and were highly viscous. This was therefore the upper limit of concentration of crude extract that could be used, but several fractions were applied at higher dose levels (CEW).

It was demonstrated in an early experiment that the activity was not abolished when aqueous solutions in the pH range from 3 to 11 were allowed to stand at room temperature for 5 days (3). This was a somewhat surprising result, because we had entertained the possibility that the active agent was phenolic and hence unstable in alkaline solution. Nevertheless, when we attempted to fractionate the crude extract with ion-exchange resins, all of the active material was lost during the experimental manipulations (3). This was shown by the loss of activity from the reconstituted fraction. Either the active material was decomposed by the extreme pH used, or else it was not eluted from one of the columns. It may have been insoluble at the extreme pH and precipitated on a column.

We next separated the extract on the basis of molecular size. For this purpose, we used a column approximately 65 cm long and 8.5 cm in diameter containing Biogel P-2, 100 to 200 mesh (BIO-RAD Laboratories). This gel has a molecular weight exclusion limit of about 1600. A 285-ml quantity of crude extract was poured on the column. Eluate samples 75 ml in volume were collected. Each sample was assayed for electrical conductivity, Cu^{++}-reducing activity (Clinitest, Ames Co.), and Ag^+ precipitability. The samples representing the large molecular weight fraction that was not retained by the gel constituted Fraction A. After this fraction passed through the column, the electrical conductance, reducing activity, and amounts of silver-precipitable material increased to peaks that nearly coincided and could not be used for separating the components of small molecular weight into clearly different fractions.

Accordingly, a separation into Fractions B and C was made between tubes containing the peak levels of reducing activity (Chart 1). This appeared to be the most reproducible point to provide a rough division of the samples. The three fractions were condensed in a flash evaporator, and final concentrations were adjusted so that equal amounts of the crude extract were represented by equal volumes of test solutions. When the various fractions, along with the starting material and the reconstituted fractions, were applied to mice, substantial activity was observed only in the starting material and the reconstituted fraction (Table 1).

Table 1

Fraction	Yield (% of crude)	Dose (CEW)		
		5	2.5	1.25
Crude			9/6[a]	1/1
A	20	0	0	0
B	49	1/1	0	0
C	32	0	0	0
Reconstituted			18/7	2/2

Activity of tobacco fractions prepared by gel filtration (A).

Thirty mice per group; all mice were treated with 125 μg of 7,12-dimethylbenz[α]anthracene (DMBA) in 0.25 ml of acetone 3 weeks prior to promotion. The experiment was terminated after 26 weeks of promoting stimulus, which consisted of daily applications of 0.25 ml of aqueous solutions. No tumors were produced by DMBA alone. DMBA followed by 0.03% croton oil in acetone produced 19 tumors in 6 mice in 10 weeks, at the end of which time this group was terminated. CEW, cigarette equivalents per week, i.e., the number of cigarettes extracted to obtain the weekly dose per mouse. The weekly dose was divided into 5 daily doses, the solvent being water.

[a]No. of tumors/No. of positive mice

It should be pointed out that in all of our studies, dilution of the starting material to half of its original concentration has nearly abolished its biologic activity. Thus a dose of 2.5 CEW has been consistently active, whereas a dose of 1.25 CEW has consistently provided an insignificant number of tumors. The

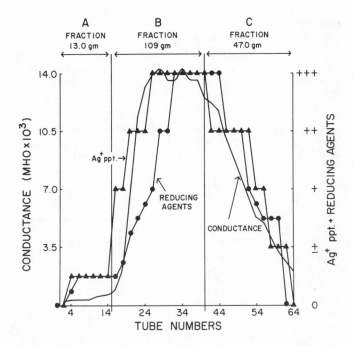

Chart 1. Typical results of gel filtration of cigarette extract. The cuts, indicated by the vertical lines, were based upon the reducing activity of the samples (see text). They varied from batch to batch by 1–2 tube numbers.

active agents of the starting material may be present just above threshold levels, so that small losses might cause negative results. In these experiments, however, Fractions A, B, and C were tested at twice the relative concentrations at which they appeared in the starting material. In view of the excellent recovery of activity in the reconstituted fraction where each of the subfractions appeared only in their starting concentration, we must conclude that none of the three fractions contained as much as half of the active agent. The active agent might have appeared at the boundary between Fractions A and B or at the boundary between Fractions B and C, under such conditions that subthreshold concentrations were somehow obtained in each of two adjoining fractions. An alternative hypothesis was that two different substances in the crude extract were both required simultaneously to exhibit biologic activity.

To decide between these hypotheses, the experiment was repeated with the additional testing of groups containing mixtures of A + B, A + C, and B + C. The results of the second experiment duplicated those of the first. The reconstituted solution was active; Fractions A, B, and C were inactive (Table 2). None of the possible combinations of two fractions contained sufficient activity to account for that of the crude starting material. Such activity as was present was generally distributed among the three different combinations. Inasmuch

Table 2

Fraction	Yield (% of crude)	Dose (CEW)		
		5	2.5	1.25
Crude			12/5[a]	1/1
A	14	0	0	
B	56	0	0	
C	30	1/1	0	
A + B			2/1	3/1
A + C			0	3/2
B + C			2/2	0
Reconstituted			13/8	5/2

Activity of tobacco fractions prepared by gel filtration (B).
Thirty mice per group treated for 26 weeks. One tumor appeared in the 7,12-dimethylbenz [α] anthracene (DMBA) controls; 240 tumors appeared in 25 tumor-bearing mice treated with DMBA followed by croton oil. CEW, cigarette equivalents per week. For explanation, see Table 1.
[a] No. of tumors/No. of positive mice.

as Groups A + B and B + C were relatively inactive, it could be concluded that a single active agent was not divided evenly by the boundary between A and B or between B and C. On the other hand, no convincing evidence of synergism was obtained.

Effect of pH. An examination of the fractions obtained during gel filtration disclosed that the starting crude extract had a pH of about 8, and Fraction A had a pH of 6.4, whereas Fractions B and C had a pH about that of the starting material. The combinations of Fraction A with either B or C had pH levels approximately equal to that of the starting material. It seemed possible that the lower pH of Fraction A might have affected the results. Accordingly, aliquots of pooled extract were adjusted to pH 7, 8, or 9 with sodium hydroxide or hydrochloric acid. The three solutions appeared to be equally active (Table 3).

Methanol Fractionation. Because aqueous solutions do not flow evenly over the skin, we were obliged to spread the extracts on the test surface. Thus the procedure was much more subjective than the simple delivery of an acetone solu-

98

tion which spreads immediately over the shaved area. We therefore spent substantial time trying to get the active material into an organic solvent. Earlier, we found that if we added acetone to the aqueous extract, the acetone-soluble fraction exhibited some activity, although not enough to account for that of the starting material (3). Using acetone in this way was also not as reproducible as we desired. Accordingly, we used methanol for this purpose.

Table 3

pH of extract	No. of tumors/No. of positive mice
7	12/3
8	14/4
9	7/3
DMBA + croton oil	42/13

Effect of pH on tumor-promoting activity of tobacco extracts. Forty mice per group treated for 35 weeks. DMBA, 7,12-dimethylbenz-[α]anthracene.

Four parts of methanol were added slowly to the crude aqueous extract with continuous stirring. The methanol-insoluble precipitate that formed was removed easily by filtration, was redissolved in water, and was treated with methanol to provide a final concentration of 80%. To all appearances, the procedure was smooth and reproducible. For the bioassay, the methanol solutions were pooled and taken to dryness on a flash evaporator. The precipitate was washed into a flask with water and then taken to dryness to remove traces of methanol. Both fractions were dissolved in water. The bioassay results were the same as those obtained by fractionation on the basis of size. The experimental manipulations caused no demonstrable loss of activity, but neither the methanol-soluble nor the methanol-insoluble fraction exhibited sufficient activity to account for that of the starting material (Table 4).

A follow-up experiment was designed to produce three fractions. Fraction D was the material insoluble in 28%

99

methanol. Fraction E contained substances soluble in 28% methanol but precipitated when the methanol concentration was raised to 95%. Fraction F consisted of substances soluble in 95% methanol. If in the earlier experiment a single agent was divided equally between the precipitate and solubles obtained with 80% methanol, the bulk of this agent should have been soluble in 28% methanol but insoluble in 95% (Fraction E). However, none of the three fractions alone was active (Table 5).

On the basis of both molecular size and methanol solubility, we concluded that the activity of alkaline aqueous extracts of unburned tobacco depends upon the simultaneous presence of

Table 4

Fraction	Yield (% of crude)	Dose (CEW)		
		5	2.5	1.25
Crude			$26/10^b$	3/3
Soluble[a]	73	3/3	0/0	
Insoluble	27	0/0	0/0	
Reconstituted			13/8	5/2

Activity of fractions prepared by methanol precipitation (A)
Thirty mice per group treated for 41 weeks. No tumors were produced by 7,12-dimethylbenz[α]anthracene (DMBA) alone; DMBA plus 0.03% croton oil in acetone produced 106 tumors in 23 positive mice. CEW, cigarette equivalents per week. For explanation, see Table 1.
[a]In 80% methanol.
[b]No. of tumors/No. of positive mice

Table 5

Fraction	Yield (% of crude)	Dose (CEW)[a]	
		5	2.5
Crude			29/12
D (least soluble)	25	0/0	1/1
E	15	1/1	0/0
F (soluble)	60	2/2	0/0
Reconstituted			53/17

Activity of fractions prepared by methanol precipitation(B).
Thirty mice per group treated for 22 weeks. No tumors were produced by 7,12-dimethylbenz [α]anthracene (DMBA) alone; DMBA + 0.03% croton oil in acetone produced 51 tumors in 11 positive mice. CEW, cigarette equivalents per week. For explanation, see Table 1.
[a]No. of tumors/No. of positive mice.

two substances, one of which is of large molecular size and hence insoluble in methanol and the other is of small molecular size and is soluble in 80% methanol.

This conclusion is being tested in an experiment that has not yet been completed. In this experiment, the extract was first treated with methanol to provide a fraction soluble in 80% methanol (M) and a methanol-insoluble fraction. The latter fraction could contain substances of large molecular weight, such as the pigments (14), and substances of small molecular weight, such as sugars and the polyhydric compounds used as humectants. The methanol-insoluble fraction was further separated by gel filtration with Biogel P-2 to provide a large molecule fraction (L) and a small molecule fraction (S). Combinations of the methanol-soluble fraction were made with the respective methanol-insoluble subfractions.

After 10 weeks, the results (Table 6) show that combinations of the methanol-soluble with either of the insoluble subfractions were active. Inasmuch as Fraction L contained only about 12% of the insoluble material, its specific activity was apparently much greater than that of Fraction S. It is again possible that a single agent was divided between L and S. If so, its molecular weight is about 1600. Alternatively, the methanol-insoluble fraction contains two or more agents of both large and small size. Only one of these agents is required to act in concert with the methanol-soluble fraction.

Tumor Promoters in Fresh Leaf. In all of the studies described thus far, we employed extracts of the tobacco obtained from a single brand of commercial cigarettes. They contained tobaccos raised in a large variety of fields under various cultural conditions. The tobacco was cured in various ways and was then further aged. Various substances, including humectants and flavoring materials, were added to the tobacco during manufacture. The tumor promoters in the final product might be an inherent characteristic of tobacco in general. Conversely, the activity of the aqueous extract might have been due to the additives, or the promoters might have been formed during aging or curing, or they might have been due to a very high level of activity produced in only a few farms, such that the final blend was active. Insecticides, for example, might be responsible for such effects.

To test these hypotheses, we extracted tobacco leaf grown in our own fields. This tobacco was raised without the use of insecticides or suckering agents. Other plants in the same field were treated by hand with DDT 7 weeks before harvest and with rotenone one week before harvest. No drifting of insecticide to the experimental plants was observed. Thus the leaf used for the studies was essentially free of nontobacco material. Immediately after picking, the leaf was ground and frozen

101

Table 6

Fraction promoting stimulus	CEW	Yield (% of crude)	No. of tumors/No. of mice
Crude	2.5		31/8
Reconstituted	2.5		26/11
M	2.5	53	0/0
S	2.5	41	0/0
L	2.5	6	0/0
M S	2.5 2.5		10/4
M S	5.0 2.5		3/3
M S	2.5 5.0		1/1
M L	2.5 2.5		3/2
M L	5.0 2.5		18/4
M L	2.5 5.0		14/4
S L	2.5 2.5		1/1
S L	2.5 5.0		0/0
S L	5.0 2.5		0/0
DMBA alone			0/0
DMBA + 0.03% croton oil			8/4

Effect of fraction recombination.
Thirty mice per group treated only 10 weeks. DMBA, 7,12-dimethylbenz-[α]anthracene; CEW, cigarette equivalents per week. For explanation, see Table 1.

to await experimental workup. Several varieties of tobacco and one variety of closely related species of Nicotiana were studied. Although direct comparisons with cigarette constituents are not possible, the amount of leaf used for each extract appears to be higher than is used for the extracts of commercial cigarettes. After 26 weeks, only the mice treated with burley extract showed any tumors. After 40 weeks, this was the only group that showed a significant tumor incidence (Table 7).

Tumor Promoters in Various Brands of Commercial Cigarettes. The precise formula used in commercial cigarettes was

Table 7

Leaf variety	Dose (gm leaf equivalent per week)	Concentration of extract (gm/ml)	No. of tumors/ No. of mice
Burley	16	0.44	6/6
Virginia	13	0.50	1/1
Canadiana	15	0.50	0
TCT	15	0.50	2/1
Nicotiniana rustica	6	0.22	1/1
Commercial cigarette	2.5 CEW		10/8
DMBA alone			1/1
DMBA + 0.03% croton oil			167/28

Tumor-promoting activity of extracts of fresh leaf.
Thirty mice per group treated for 40 weeks. DMBA, 7,12-dimethylbenz(a)anthracene: CEW, cigarette equivalents per week. For explanation, see Table 1.

not available to us. Many of the constituents are known generally in the industry, but specific ingredients may remain a trade secret. In order to determine whether the activity of the commercial extract was due to a unique constituent of that particular brand, cigarettes of five American and two English companies were studied. The American cigarettes were all typical blends primarily of burley and bright tobaccos; the English brands contained bright tobaccos. A pilot study showed that some of the samples were toxic when applied at a dose of 2.5 CEW. The toxicity seemed to be related to the pH of the extract. Accordingly, the extracts were all treated with HCl to provide a final pH of 7.1 to 7.3 and were adjusted to a concentration of 0.8 gm of solids per milliliter. The treated extracts were tolerated reasonably well by the experimental animals.

All of the brands yielded active extracts (Table 8). It is apparent that no unique formula used by any particular cigarette manufacturer accounted for the results observed in these experiments. It is also obvious that cigarettes made of all bright tobacco contain tumor promoters, just as do cigarettes which are made of a blend of bright and burley tobaccos. The significance of the earlier experiment with fresh leaf in which only burley tobacco gave measurable activity is thus somewhat in question.

Comparison with Data Obtained by Other Investigators. Tumorigenic activity in extracts of unburned tobacco have been reported a number of times (8, 10, 17, 20). Van Duuren et al. (17) characterized the tumor promoters of unburned tobacco by extracting the tobacco with a series of solvents of increasing polarity. They observed activity in the less polar fractions. Similar results are being obtained in a study we are conducting in collaboration with Dr. O. T. Chortyk.[3] The slightly polar promoting agents differ from the ones that I have discussed in the present account in regard to solubility and in their ability to act alone in mice treated with DMBA.

Table 8

Brand[a]	No. of mice alive at 7th week	No. of tumors/ No. of mice
A	45	75/21
B	46	33/15
C	45	47/20
D	49	10/9
E	46	54/10
F	50	21/7
G	47	46/17
DMBA alone	41	0/0
DMBA + 0.03% croton oil	49	274/29

Tumor promoters in various brands of commercial cigarettes.
Fifty mice per group treated for 26 weeks; extract concentrations were 0.8 gm/ml.

[a]Brands A through E were blended U.S. cigarettes; F and G were English cigarettes consisting of bright tobacco.

[3]Unpublished observation from a study carried out under contract with the Agricultural Research Service, U. S. Department of Agriculture, administered by the Eastern Utilization Research and Development Division, 600 East Mermaid Lane, Philadelphia, Pennsylvania 19118.

ACKNOWLEDGMENTS

Miss Helen Fox, Dr. Yasushi Kodama, Mr. Huston Myers and Miss Maryama Ramadhan were of great assistance in carrying out the technical parts of these studies. The fresh leaf was grown under the direction of Dr. Seaward A. Sand.

REFERENCES

1. Atkinson, L., Chester, I. C., Smyth, F. G., and ten Seldam, R. E. J. Oral Cancer in New Guinea. A Study in Demography and Etiology. Cancer, *17:* 1289–1298, 1964.
2. Bock, F. G., Moore, G. E., and Crouch, S. K. Tumor-promoting Activity of Extracts of Unburned Tobacco. Science, *145:* 831–833, 1964.
3. Bock, F. G., Shamberger, R. J., and Myers, H. K. Tumour-promoting Agents in Unburned Cigarette Tobacco. Nature, *208:* 584–585, 1965.
4. Chang, K. M. Experimental Production of Lesions on Cheek Pouch of the Hamster by Betel Quid. J. Formosan Med. Assoc., *65:* 125–131, 1966.
5. Davis, G. G. Buyo Cheek Cancer with Special Reference to Etiology. J. Am. Med. Assoc., *64:* 711–718, 1915.
6. Doll, R. Interpretations of Epidemiologic Data. Cancer Res., *23:* 1613–1623, 1963.
7. Moore, G. E., Bissinger, L. L., and Proehl, E. C. Intraoral Cancer and the Use of Chewing Tobacco, J. Am. Geriat. Soc., *1:* 497–505, 1953.
8. Muir, C. S., and Kirk, R. Betel, Tobacco, and Cancer of the Mouth. Brit. J. Cancer, *14:* 597–608, 1960.
9. Orr, I. M. Oral Cancer in Betel Nut Chewers in Travancore. Lancet, *2:* 575–580, 1933.
10. Ranadive, K. J., Gothoskar, S. V., and Khanolkar, V. R. Experimental Studies on the Etiology of Cancer Types Specific to India (a) Oral Cancer (b) Kangri Cancer. Acta Unio Intern. Contra Cancrum, *19:* 634–639. 1963.
11. Roe, F. J. C., Salaman, M. H., and Cohen, J. Incomplete Carcinogens in Cigarette Smoke Condensate. Tumor-promotion by a Phenolic Fraction. Brit. J. Cancer, *3:* 623–633, 1959.
12. Rosenfeld, L., and Callaway, J. Snuff Dippers Cancer. Am. J. Surg., *106:* 840–844, 1963.
13. Singh, A. D., and Von Essen, C. F. Buccal Mucosa Cancer in South India. Etiologic and Clinical Aspects. Am. J. Roentgenol, Radium Therapy Nucl. Med., *96:* 6–14, 1966.
14. Stedman, R. L. Chemical Composition of Tobacco and Tobacco Smoke. Chem. Rev., *68:* 153–207, 1968.
15. U.S. Public Health Service, Smoking and Health. Washington, D.C.: U.S. Government Printing Office, Publication No. 1103, 1964.
16. U.S. Public Health Service, The Health Consequences of Smoking. A Public Health Service Review: 1967. Washington, D. C.: U. S. Government Printing Office, Publication No. 1696, 1967.

17. Van Duuren, B. L., Sivak, A., Segal, A., Orriš, L., and Langseth, L. The Tumor-Promoting Agents of Tobacco Leaf and Tobacco Smoke Condensate. J. Natl. Cancer Inst., *37:* 519–526, 1966.
18. Wynder, E. L., and Hoffmann, D. A Study of Tobacco Carcinogenesis. VIII. The Role of the Acidic Fractions as Promoters. Cancer, *14:* 1306–1315, 1961.
19. Wynder, E. L., and Hoffmann, D. Tobacco and Tobacco Smoke. Studies in Experimental Carcinogenesis. New York: Academic Press, 1968.
20. Wynder, E. L., and Wright, G. A Study of Tobacco Carcinogenesis. I. The Primary Fractions. Cancer, *10:* 255–271, 1957.

A STUDY OF TOBACCO CARCINOGENESIS
X. *Tumor Promoting Activity*

Ernest L. Wynder, MD, and Dietrich Hoffmann, PhD

Tobacco smoke condensate is carcinogenic to several animal species and a variety of animal tissues.[25, 26] This effect is in part due to carcinogenic polynuclear aromatic hydrocarbons (PAH). The role of PAH seems to be principally that of a tumor initiator and therefore the total carcinogenic activity of tobacco smoke condensate must relate partly to tumor promoting or cocarcinogenic factors. We use the term promoter when an agent is applied to mouse skin days after tumor initiation. Cocarcinogens not only evoke (promote) dormant (initiated) tumor cells but may also condition the tumorigenic effects of carcinogens ranging from merely facilitating the absorption of compounds to enhancing the activity of a carcinogen by chemical and/or biochemical interactions.

Among the hundreds of different structures of constituents of tobacco smoke condensate, these might well include a variety of cocarcinogenic factors. For this reason, it may be difficult to fully explain the promoting and/or cocarcinogenic effects of a particular tobacco smoke condensate. The present study has been aimed at investigating the promoting activity of various tobacco and non-tobacco smoke condensates as well as tobacco extracts.

PREVIOUS STUDIES

Certain tobacco extracts and smoke condensates are known to promote tumors on mouse skin previously initiated with a subthreshold dose of a carcinogen (Table 1). Gellhorn[6] has shown that mice initiated with 200 µg of benzo(a)pyrene (BaP) and subsequently receiving topical application of a solution of 10% cigarette smoke condensate 3 times a week, developed significantly more tumors than upon applying either the carcinogen or the condensate alone. A tumor-promoting effect is also observed on mouse skin initiated with 75, 150, or 300 µg of 7, 12-dimethylbenz(a)anthracene (DMBA) and then treated 3 times a week with a 50% "tar" suspension in acetone.[1, 18, 19, 22] The findings by Van Duuren et al. and by Bock[1, 18, 20] that tobacco extracts have tumor-promoting activity, gain importance because the activity of smoke condensate as a complete carcinogen is significantly greater than that of tobacco extracts.[25] Fractions of tobacco extracts have been tested as tumor promoters only to a limited extent, but promoting activity has been demonstrated for the strong and weakly acidic and neutral portions of cigarette smoke condensate.[2, 16, 22, 25]

Bock et al., as well as Van Duuren et al., showed that a barium hydroxide extract of tobacco had tumor-promoting activity.[1, 20] However, since chemical changes are likely

From the Division of Environmental Cancerigenesis, Sloan-Kettering Institute for Cancer Research, New York, N.Y.

Supported by American Cancer Society Grant E-231 and in part by National Cancer Institute Grant CA-08748.

The authors wish to acknowledge the excellent assistance of Mrs. B. Stahl-Rathkamp.

TABLE 1. Experiments on Tobacco Products as Tumor Promoters

Investigator & study	Preparation of material	Biological procedure (I-Initiation and P-Promotion)	Results
Gwynn & Salaman 1953 Tobacco extract	Methanol extract of whole unburned (Virginia) cigs.	(I) 0.15% DMBA (P) Extract applied for 23 weeks (4.5% conc.)	No tumors
Gwynn 1954 Extracts of butts of Virginian & Rhodesian cigs.	Butts dried and extracted in a soxhlet with methanol for 1 hr. 40% of butt wt. extracted.	(I) Single dose DMBA (P) 5% sol. of extract bi-weekly for 161 days.	No tumors
Gwynn & Salaman 1956 Smoke condensate of British Virginia & American tobaccos, I & II.	Condensate obtained from smoking machines which simulated normal smoking conditions.	(I) Single 0.2 ml dose, 0.15% DMBA (P) 0.06 ml tar diluted 3–5 times with acetone was applied once/twice a week. 20 "S" stock mice/group.	In one tar group: squamous ca in 2 mice, in 25th week. No others noted.
Hamer & Woodhouse 1956 Smoke condensate from British cigs.	Cigs. smoked in glass apparatus by alternating suction. Smoke collected in 4 acetone traps.	(I) 3 × 0.3% BaP in acetone (P) 20% tar solution (60 mg/mouse) twice a week for 18 months 30 outbred strain albino mice	Four mice with papillomas. Weak tumor-promoting activity. No paps. in BaP control group.
Gellhorn 1958 Cigarette smoke condensate	Loose tobacco burned in 2.5 diam. cylinder of all-glass smoking machine. Collection in 6 alcohol-CO₂ traps.	(I) 200 µg BaP/daily for 2 days. (P) Tobacco tar applied in acetone or benzene interscapulary 5–6 times/week. av. application 10 mg tar.	Study: 581 mice: 35 with ca.; 61 with paps. Control: BaP only—529 mice: 17 ca.; 20 paps. Tar only: (595 mice) 2 ca., 10 paps.
Roe et al. 1959 Phenolic fraction of cig. smoke condensate from British cigs.	Smoke cond. from 1000 cigs. at a time smoked in automatic machine, collected in CO₂-acetone traps.	(I) 0.2 ml of 0.15% DMBA acetone. Single dose. (P) 3× weekly for 40 weeks. Applications varied 12.5% – 25% of phenolic fraction 110 inbred strain ♂ and ♀ mice	DMBA + Promoter (30 mice): 1 with ca.; 15 with 65 papillomas. Promoter only (30 mice): no ca., no papillomas DMBA only (50 mice): no ca., 4 with 6 paps.
Clemo & Miller 1960 Neutral fraction of cig. smoke condensate	12 cigs. smoked in an apparatus to simulate average natural smoking. The non-volatiles trapped in methanol (6.8g from 100 g tobacco) and fractionated. The neutral portion was used as promoter.	(I) Fraction of city smoke containing PAH applied 3× weekly for 2 weeks. (P) Three weeks after initiation neutral portion of "tar" applied 3× weekly until death.	I + P: 21 mice, 1 with ca., 3 with 4 paps. I alone: 21 mice, 3 with ca., 12 with 17 paps. C57B1 mice, 3-6 weeks.
Wynder & Hoffmann 1961 Acidic & phenolic fractions of cigarette smoke condensate.	85 mm cigarettes smoked on smoking machine and condensate collected in cold traps.	(I) 75 µg DMBA in single doses. (P) 12 months of application of "tar" (50%). Phenolic fraction (5%, 10% + 25%), and acidic fractions (10%) were applied.	DMBA only: 7% w/ca., 10% w/paps. DMBA + Tar(2× weekly): 27% w/ca. 43% w/paps. DMBA + Tar(3×weekly): 37% w/ca. 63% w/paps. DMBA + 10% phenolic frac. (3× weekly): no. ca., 30% w/paps. DMBA + 25% phenolic frac.(3× weekly):3%w/ca. 53% w/paps.
		Comparison: BaP solution (0.005%) painted 3× weekly (total dose: 750 µg per mouse). Tar (50%), phenolic frac. (5%, 10%, and 25%), and acidic frac. (10%) applied for 12 months. 30 Ha/ICR Mil. Swiss Albino 8-9 weeks old female mice.	BaP (3× weekly): 68% w/ca., 70% w/paps. BaP (3× weekly) + 5% phenolic (2× weekly): 93% w/ca., 77% w/paps. BaP (3× weekly) + 10% phenolic (2× weekly): 97% w/ca., 93% w/paps. BaP (3× weekly) + 10% acidic (2× weekly): 93% w/ca., 80% w/paps.

TABLE 1 (*Continued*)

Investigator & study	Preparation of material	Biological procedure (I-Initiation and P-Promotion)	Results
Guérin 1961 Smoke condensate of French cigarettes	Automatic smoking machine	(I) BaP, 0.25ml of 1% soln. applied once weekly for 4 weeks (total dose: 10 mg) (P) "Tar" from 2 cigs. painted once weekly for 4 weeks, twice weekly for 4 weeks and 3✕ weekly thereafter. 3 groups of 80 mice. Ha/ICR Mil. Swiss Albino 8–9 weeks old female mice.	BaP + "tar"—69 survivors; 57.9% with skin tumors. "tar" alone—79 survivors; 20.2% with skin tumors. BaP alone—63 survivors; 22% with skin tumors.
Ranadive et al. 1963 Extract of "Vadakan" Indian tobacco	Tobacco was powdered, treated with 2% HCl for removal of alkaloids and extracted with acetone.	(I) Single painting of "microdose" of BaP to two groups of mice: A and B. Single application of BaP, then bi-weekly application of extract for 80 weeks. Mice: Group A: Swiss Albino. Group B: Swiss Albino (hairless mice)	*BaP* A: No tumors after 80 weeks (7 mice) *BaP* B: Slight epid. hyperplasia in 2 out of 10 mice. *BaP + Extract* A: 1 pap. (16 mice) *BaP + Extract* B: 1 pap., 1 epid. after 41 weeks (13 mice), 3 squamous paps., 1 basal cell ca. after 80 weeks.
Bock et al. 1964 Extract of cigarette tobacco	Test solutions: 1. Tobacco extracted twice with acetone. Residue extracted with benzene, & concentrate (15–29g) dissolved in acetone to vol. of 40 ml. 2. Tobacco treated with aqueous Ba(OH)₂. Mixture filtered, residue extracted twice with dist. H₂O; BaCO₃ removed. 3. Tobacco treated with aqueous Ba(OH)₂ and then neutralized.	(I) 125 μg DMBA in 25 ml acetone applications. (P) 3 weeks later: .25 ml test solution applied 5✕ weekly. 3 test 30 female Swiss ICR hairless mice per group.	All extracts had tumor promoting activity; at 36th week. Test soln. (1): 7 mice with 16 tumors. Test soln. (2): 8 mice with 20 tumors Test soln. (3): Control— 2 mice with 11 tumors Control: no paps.
Van Duuren et al. 1966 Flue cured tobacco	Powdered tobacco leaf placed in soxhlet and extractions made of test solutions (1): methyl-alcohol, (2) ether, (3) chloroform. Also tested (4) reconstituted tobacco extract and (5) cigarette smoke condensate.	(I) DMBA (150 μg) in 0.1 ml acetone applied once. (P) Extracts applied 3✕ weekly for 12–14 months 20 Ha/ICR/Mil. Swiss Albino female mice in each group.	Test soln. (1): 13 mice with 2 paps; 2 ca. Test soln. (2): 12 mice with 1 pap., no ca. Test soln. (3): 10 mice with 1 pap; no ca. Test soln. (4): 14 mice with 5 paps; no ca. Test soln. (5): 10 mice with 11 paps; 4 ca.
Van Duuren et al. 1967 Whole tobacco extract (WTE) Whole cigarette condensate (WCE)	See Van Duuren et al 1966	(I) DMBA subcutaneous (sc) and intraperitoneal (ip) injections; 500 μg BaP, ip; Solvent: tricapylin. 20 mg Urethane (U) sc + ip; Solvent: saline (P) 25 mg WTE or WCE, 3✕ wkly. 20 Ha/ICR/Mil Swiss albino female mice per group.	500 μg sc + WTE: 2 mice w/paps; 5 tumors 50 μg DMBA sc + WTE: 1 mouse with pap; 1 tumor U sc + WCT: 3 mice with paps; 3 w/tumor 500 μg DMBA ip + WCT: 4 mice w/paps; 6 tumors. U ip + WCT: No mice with paps; no tumors BaP ip + WTE: No mice w/paps. No tumors BaP ip + WCT: 2 mice w/paps; 2 tumors Controls: No paps., no tumors. (initiator alone)

TABLE 1. (Continued)

Investigation & study	Preparation of material	Biological procedure (I-Initiation and P-Promotion)	Results
Van Duuren et al. 1968 Barium hydroxide (Ba(OH)₂) and acetone-benzene extracts of tobacco.	"Extract" preparations, see Bock et al. 1964	(I) Single DMBA dose (150μg) in 10μl acetone. (P) 3× weekly (a) 8 mg Ba(OH)₂ extract in 100 μl water; (b) 50 mg acetone-benzene extract in 100 μl acetone. Prom. application: 1 year. Each group: 20 Ha/ ICR/Mil. Swiss Albino female mice.	DMBA + Ba(OH)₂ extract: 6 mice w/paps; 1 ca. DMBA + acetone-benzene extract: 2 mice with paps; no ca. Ba(OH)₂ extract: no mice with paps; no ca. Acetone-benzene extract: no paps; no ca. DMBA alone: 2 mice with paps; 1 ca.

to occur during such treatment, evaluation of these experiments is difficult. Some volatile phenols possess tumor-promoting activity. Their partial or even nearly complete elimination from tobacco smoke by filtration, however, has not reduced the tumorigenicity of the resulting "tar."[25]*

At present, we know of no single component nor of a single class of components that is solely or even primarily responsible for the established tumor-promoting activity of tobacco "tar" or of tobacco extracts.

METHODS AND MATERIALS

Tobacco smoke condensates: All tobacco and non-tobacco "tars" used in this study were obtained, prepared, and stored in a standardized manner.[25]

Smoke condensates of non-tobacco cigarettes: The non-tobacco cigarettes (85 mm straights) were produced from Lespedeza hay and fresh spinach. The hay was purchased from a farmer in North Carolina. The spinach was purchased through a produce broker and was delivered from Texas in the usual crates packed with ice.

The spinach was dried from approximately 90% moisture to approximately 15% moisture by spreading it on racks in a drying room maintained at 37°C. It was then cut on a Himhoff cutter at 30 cuts/inch and made into cigarettes using an AMF cigarette-making machine. The cigarettes produced were

of poor quality due to the brittle nature of the dried spinach which tended to disintegrate very easily into fines. The yield of usable cigarettes was approximately 400 cigarettes per 100 pounds of fresh spinach. A sample was submitted for routine "tar" analysis. The "tar" yield of mg/cig. has a wide experimental deviation (± 20%) due to extreme difficulty in keeping the cigarettes lighted between puffs.

The hay was converted into 85 mm straight cigarettes by first passing it through a hammer mill having a ½" mesh basket to reduce its size and then producing cigarettes on an AMF cigarette-making machine. The "tar" yield was 25.1 mg/cig.

These cigarettes were smoked on a 100 unit smoker.[25] The cigarette paper used on both samples was Schweitzer's 136-1.

Tobacco extracts: Batches of 250 g of Turkish tobacco were extracted with 1250 ml distilled dimethylsulfoxide (DMSO) at 60°C for 3 hours. The resulting extract was suction-filtered and the solvent extraction repeated twice. All extracts were combined and the excess DMSO distilled off at a water bath temperature of 65–70°C/1 mm Hg until a concentration of about 50% (w/v) solution could be determined for an aliquot. An exact 50% solution was then prepared for biologic testing. Each 100 g of tobacco yielded about 60 g of extract.

Bioassays: Six-week old HA/ICR/Mil (Swiss Albino) female mice were used and the test started in the second telogen phase of the hair cycle (7–8 weeks). Each animal received by pipette a single dose of either 150 or 300 μg DMBA (freshly purified) in

---

* Throughout the paper the term "tar" is used for convenience only, although it is not correct physiochemically.

50 μl acetone (spectra grade quality) on the shaved skin of the back. The application of tobacco "tars" or extracts began 10 days later. Solutions .were painted with Camel hair brushes (No. 5) thrice weekly for 12 months. The average "tar" dose applied with a 50% tobacco smoke condensate acetone suspension is 75 mg (average from 40 applications). Surviving animals were observed without further treatment for another 2 months and then killed. All tumors which had attained a diameter of 1 mm and which did not regress for 21 consecutive days were recorded. When an epithelioma was grossly recognized, animals were autopsied and appropriate histologic sections taken.

RESULTS

Table 2 summarizes the effect of initiating doses of 150 μg and 300 μg of DMBA on the tumor promotion by standard cigarette smoke condensate.[25] Tumors occur significantly earlier in animals initiated with the 300 μg dose in terms of percent tumor-bearing mice as well as total number of papillomas. After 5 months of application of the tumor promoter ("tar"), for example, in the 150 μg group only one mouse had a single tumor while 10 mice had a total of 13 tumors in the high dosage group (P < 0.01). At 9 months, twice as many tumors were observed in the high initiator dose group as in the low initiator dose group; the former group also containing 5 mice with 6 carcinomas

compared with one carcinoma in the low dosage group. At 14 months, however, the tumor yield is comparable in the 2 groups (P > 0.05). Thus, a higher initiation dose appears to shorten the latency period and invoke a greater number of tumors earlier although the final tumor yield is comparable for both initiation doses.

Difference in tobacco types: The tumor-promoting effects of condensates from cigarettes made of flue- and air-cured tobaccos are compared in Table 3. The toxicity of the condensates was reflected in the high mortality during the first months. This aspect needs to be considered when the tumor yield in this experiment is compared with other results. The experiment does afford comparison of all Burley and Bright tobaccos in which the promoting activity appears to be similar. Tests for complete carcinogenicity of cigarette smoke condensates from these 2 types had previously revealed significant differences.[23]

Tobacco cuts and tobacco stems: Table 4 presents experiments comparing the tumor-promoting activity of "tars" from a standard tobacco blend with cuts of 20 and 50 times per inch (normal cut: 30/inch). Again, animals were initiated with doses of 150 μg and 300 μg DMBA. Since there were no significant differences between these "tars" with either initiating dose, we present only the results with the lower dose of DMBA. This result parallels the earlier reported data on the complete carcinogenicity of "tars" from cigarettes

TABLE 2. Effect of Initiating Dose on Tumor Promotion Activity of Cigarette Smoke Condensate
Experiment I: DMBA (300 μg) + 50% smoke condensate from cigarettes with standard tobacco blend (30 cuts/inch)
Experiment II: DMBA (150 μg) + 50% smoke condensate from cigarettes with standard tobacco blend (30 cuts/inch)

Months	Surviving mice I	II	No. of mice with papillomas (Total no. of papillomas) I	II	No. of mice with carcinoma (Total no. of carcinomas) I	II
1	60	60				
2	60	60	3 (3)	—	—	—
3	58	60	4 (4)	—	—	—
4	57	60	7 (8)	—	—	—
5	52	58	10 (13)	1 (1)	1 (1)	—
6	51	54	10 (13)	3 (4)	2 (2)	—
7	48	54	11 (15)	6 (7)	2 (2)	—
8	43	53	12 (20)	7 (9)	3 (3)	—
9	37	52	16 (42)	11 (21)	5 (6)	1 (1)
10	33	45	20 (46)	15 (29)	6 (6)	2 (2)
11	29	42	21 (48)	15 (29)	6 (6)	2 (2)
12	25	39	23 (50)	17 (31)	8 (8)	5 (5)
13	15	37	25 (52)	21 (35)	9 (9)	7 (7)
14	8	25	26 (55)	26 (51)	9 (9)	7 (7)

Each group was started with 60 mice.

TABLE 3.
Experiment I:—150 μg DMBA + 50% smoke condensate from cigarettes with Burley tobacco
Experiment II:—150 μg DMBA + 50% smoke condensate from cigarettes with Bright tobacco

Months	Surviving mice		Number of mice with papillomas (total no. of papillomas)		Number of mice with carcinoma (total number of carcinomas)	
	I	II	I	II	I	II
1	34	37	—	—	—	—
2	32	37	—	—	—	—
3	30	36	—	—	—	—
4	28	34	—	—	—	—
5	26	34	1 (1)	2 (2)	—	—
6	25	28	1 (1)	2 (2)	—	—
7	24	28	2 (2)	2 (2)	—	—
8	24	28	3 (3)	3 (3)	—	—
9	22	28	5 (7)	6 (6)	—	—
10	21	26	6 (9)	9 (12)	—	—
11	19	26	9 (13)	10 (13)	—	—
12	19	26	12 (19)	10 (15)	2 (2)	—
13	17	25	12 (19)	10 (16)	2 (2)	1 (1)
14	17	25	12 (20)	10 (17)	4 (4)	3 (3)

Each group was started with 50 mice.

made from the same tobacco blend but differet cuts.[24]

"Tars" obtained from cigarettes made exclusively of tobacco stems were significantly lower in tumor-promoting activity (P < 0.01). This is reflected both by the number of animals with tumors and the total tumor yield (Table 5). We repeated this experiment by applying the "tars" in concentrations of 33% and 50% on mouse skin initiated with 150 μg DMBA. Again we observed a lower papilloma yield among mice that had received the "tar" from cigarettes made entirely from stems. The tumor-promoting activities of the 33% and 50% condensates of stems were significantly lower than

the corresponding concentrations of standard "tars" (P < 0.01), Fig. 1. Since, as shown in a previous experiment, a 50% "stem tar" produced as complete carcinogen only 7 tumor-bearing mice in a group of 50 (14%) and on mouse skin initiated with 150 μg DMBA only 16 tumor-bearing mice in a group of 90 (18%), we did in fact not establish any tumor-promoting activity for the stem "tar." In comparison, our current tests (1965–68) for standard "tar" showed a 20% tumor yield (30 out of 150 mice) when tested as complete carcinogen and a 39% tumor yield (35 out of 90 mice) on skin initiated with 150 μg DMBA.

Tobacco additives: We tested "tars" ob-

TABLE 4.
Experiment I: 150 μg DMBA + 50% smoke condensate from cigarettes with standard tobacco blend (coarse cut; 20 cuts/inch)
Experiment II: 150 μg DMBA + 50% smoke condensate from cigarettes with standard tobacco blend (fine cut; 50 cuts/inch)

Months	Surviving mice		No. of mice with papillomas (total no. of papillomas)		No. of mice with carcinoma (total no. of carcinomas)	
	I	II	I	II	I	II
1	50	50	—	—	—	—
2	49	50	—	—	—	—
3	49	47	—	—	—	—
4	48	46	—	—	—	—
5	48	44	—	—	—	—
6	48	44	—	—	—	—
7	48	43	6 (6)	1 (1)	—	—
8	47	42	7 (7)	3 (5)	—	—
9	45	41	8 (13)	6 (11)	—	—
10	43	40	10 (22)	7 (14)	—	—
11	40	40	15 (32)	14 (28)	—	—
12	40	36	15 (38)	14 (31)	2 (2)	—
13	36	35	17 (40)	14 (34)	3 (3)	1 (1)
14	32	31	21 (44)	17 (37)	7 (7)	5 (5)

Each group was started with 50 mice.

112

TABLE 5.

Experiment IV: 150 µg DMBA + 50% smoke condensate from cigarettes from stems for
standard tobacco blend
Experiment V: 150 µg DMBA + 50% smoke condensate from cigarettes from standard
tobacco blend

Months	Surviving mice		No. of mice with papillomas (total no. of papillomas)		No. of mice with carcinoma (total no. of carcinomas)	
	IV	V	IV	V	IV	V
1	60	60	—	—	—	—
2	60	60	—	—	—	—
3	57	60	1 (1)	—	—	—
4	57	60	1 (1)	—	—	—
5	56	58	1 (1)	1 (1)	—	—
6	56	54	1 (1)	3 (4)	—	—
7	49	54	3 (3)	6 (7)	—	—
8	48	53	5 (5)	7 (9)	—	—
9	48	52	6 (6)	11 (21)	—	2 (2)
10	48	45	7 (7)	15 (29)	1 (1)	2 (2)
11	48	42	8 (8)	15 (29)	1 (1)	5 (5)
12	48	39	8 (8)	17 (31)	1 (1)	7 (7)
13	46	37	10 (10)	21 (35)	1 (1)	7 (7)
14	46	25	10 (10)	26 (51)	—	—

Each group was started with 60 mice.

tained from 2 groups of cigarettes in which 8.3% sodium nitrate or 5% copper (II) nitrate had been added to the standard tobacco. Table 6 shows the promoting effect of these "tars" on mouse epithelium initiated with 300 µg DMBA. There is no significant difference between the number of tumor-bearing mice in the promoting activity of "tars" from the additive cigarettes and control cigarettes. However, differences became apparent in respect to a greater multiplicity of tumors on animals treated with the control "tar." The latter aspects become apparent also when the tumor-promoting activity of standard "tar" and "tar" from Cu (NO₃)₂ cigarettes is compared on mouse skin initiated with 150 µg DMBA (Table 7). As for the standard "tar," the promoting activity of "tar" from Cu (NO₃)₂ cigarettes is comparable when applied to skin initiated with 150 µg or 300 µg DMBA.

Tobacco substitutes: The promoting activity of "tars" obtained from cigarettes made of spinach and hay (Table 8) is compared with that of standard cigarettes (Table 2). In mice treated with DMBA and "tar" from hay cigarettes, tumors appeared later and are fewer than in a control group receiving DMBA and cigarette smoke condensate. The tumor-promoting activity of spinach "tar" was similar to that of tobacco "tar."

In evaluating the hay "tar" experiment, we must allow for an interruption in the seventh month due to exhaustion of test materials. Six applications were mixed at that time but were added to the regular schedule

after painting was resumed. We believe that this incident had no effect on the conclusion that hay "tar" has a significantly lower promoting activity than tobacco "tar."

For better evaluation of the tumor-promoting activity of spinach "tar," one should test this tar for complete carcinogenic activity. The difficulty and cost of preparing the number of cigarettes required in such an experiment prevented our carrying out this test. Such a test conducted with hay "tar" showed

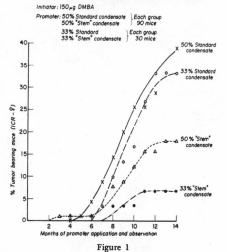

TUMOR PROMOTING ACTIVITIES OF CIGARETTE SMOKE CONDENSATE

Figure 1

113

TABLE 6.

Experiment I: 300 μg DMBA + 50% smoke condensate from cigarettes with standard tobacco with 8.3% NaNO₃

Experiment II: 300 μg DMBA + 50% smoke condensate from cigarettes with standard tobacco with 5% Cu(NO₃)₂

Months	Surviving mice I	II	No. of mice with papillomas (total number of papillomas) I	II	No. of mice with carcinoma (total number of carcinomas) I	II
1	59	59	1 (2)	3 (4)	—	—
2	56	58	2 (3)	4 (6)	—	—
3	55	56	3 (4)	4 (7)	—	—
4	49	50	4 (5)	4 (7)	—	—
5	47	50	8 (9)	7 (10)	—	—
6	47	50	10 (11)	8 (11)	1 (2)	—
7	46	50	10 (11)	8 (11)	1 (2)	—
8	45	47	11 (12)	11 (14)	2 (3)	1 (1)
9	43	46	14 (15)	12 (16)	3 (4)	1 (1)
10	41	45	15 (17)	13 (17)	3 (4)	1 (1)
11	39	43	19 (21)	15 (19)	4 (5)	2 (2)
12	33	42	19 (21)	16 (20)	4 (5)	2 (2)
13	32	40	21 (23)	17 (21)	5 (6)	3 (3)
14	24	40	21 (24)	17 (21)	6 (7)	3 (3)

Each group was started with 60 mice.

very low carcinogenicity. For this test, 100 mice were painted with a 50% hay "tar" in acetone suspension for 15 months and the surviving mice observed for another 3 months. Only 2 mice developed one tumor each; both were carcinomas.

When dealing with the tobacco substitutes, the difficulties involved in smoking the materials in a standardized manner must be considered. Although it has been attempted to have the same width of cut and moisture content as obtained with tobacco cigarettes, some differences in burning characteristics remain, which affect the chemical and physicochemical processes during combustion.

Tobacco extracts: A comparison of the tumor-promoting activity of a DMSO extract of Turkish tobacco with that of tobacco smoke condensate is presented in Table 9. The DMSO controls gave 4 tumor-bearing mice from a group of 60 mice. Since, in our experience, up to 5% of the mice receiving 150 μg of DMBA as initiator may develop papillomas, the tumors obtained in the DMSO control are not inidicative of promoting activity for the solvent. The DMSO extract of tobacco tested on mouse skin without DMBA initiation produced only one tumor in a group of 50 mice after 14 months. We applied on the average the same amount of material as we

TABLE 7.

Experiment I: 150 μg DMBA + 50% smoke condensate from cigarettes with standard tobacco with 5% Cu(NO₃)₂

Experiment II: 150 μg DMBA + 50% smoke condensate from cigarettes with standard tobacco blend

Months	Surviving mice I	II	No. of mice with papillomas (total no. of papillomas) I	II	No. of mice with carcinoma (total no. of carcinomas) I	II
1	49	60	—	—	—	—
2	47	60	1 (1)	—	—	—
3	47	60	1 (1)	—	—	—
4	46	60	1 (1)	—	—	—
5	45	58	1 (1)	1 (1)	—	—
6	42	54	1 (1)	3 (4)	—	—
7	40	54	1 (1)	6 (7)	—	—
8	40	53	3 (3)	7 (9)	—	—
9	38	52	6 (7)	11 (21)	—	1 (1)
10	38	45	8 (9)	15 (29)	—	2 (2)
11	37	42	9 (11)	15 (29)	1 (1)	2 (2)
12	35	39	15 (19)	17 (31)	2 (2)	5 (5)
13	32	37	17 (21)	21 (35)	4 (4)	7 (7)
14	29	25	20 (24)	26 (51)	7 (7)	7 (7)

Group I was started with 50 mice.
Group II was started with 60 mice.

TABLE 8.
Experiment I: 150 µg DMBA + 50% smoke condensate from cigarettes made from hay
Experiment II: 150 µg DMBA + 50% smoke condensate from cigarettes made from spinach

Months	Surviving mice I	II	No. of mice with papillomas (total no. of papillomas) I	II	No. of mice with carcinoma (total no. of carcinomas) I	II
1	50	50	—	—	—	—
2	50	47	—	—	—	—
3	50	45	—	—	—	—
4	49	45	—	—	—	—
5	46	45	—	—	—	—
6	45	44	2(2)	—	—	—
7	45	44	4(4)	—	—	—
8	44	40	4(4)	1(1)	—	1(1)
9	43	37	6(6)	3(4)	—	1(1)
10	40	31	6(6)	11(18)	—	1(1)
11	38	31	8(8)	14(25)	—	2(2)
12	37	25	9(10)	15(29)	1(1)	3(3)
13	36	22	10(11)	16(32)	1(1)	3(3)
14	33	21	10(11)	16(32)	1(1)	3(3)

Each group was started with 50 mice.

applied for smoke condensate (75 mg with each painting).

The promoting effects for the DMSO extract of the Turkish tobacco and for the tobacco smoke condensate, however, are apparently similar. In a short-term test, the extract showed no hyperplasia and sebaceous gland destruction in contrast to the effects of tobacco smoke condensate.

The evaluation of such findings requires several considerations. As stated, DMSO extraction of 100 g of tobacco yields 60 g of residual material. The condensate of the mainstream smoke of a cigarette equals about 3% of the weight of the tobacco which is burned from the first puff until a butt length of 23 mm. About twice this amount is contained in the side-stream smoke condensate which is not included in our test material. Furthermore, one needs to take into account the possible effect of tobacco combustion on the destruction and/or synthesis of carcinogenic factors.

The fact that significant tumor-promoting activity has been demonstrated for the DMSO extract of Turkish tobacco suggests there may be at least one type of tumor promoter in tobacco smoke condensate which has not resulted from the combustion process alone.

Benzo(a)pyrene and phenol data: The benzo(a)pyrene and phenol values for a number of the materials tested in this study are given in Table 10. While previous investigations indicated that these values were re-

TABLE 9.
Experiment I: 150 µg DMBA + 50% DMSO extract of Turkish tobacco
Experiment II: 150 µg DMBA + 50% smoke condensate from cigarettes with standard tobacco blend

Months	Surviving mice I	II	Number of mice with papillomas (total no. of papillomas) I	II	Number of mice with carcinoma (total no. of carcinomas) I	II
1	60	60	—	—	—	—
2	60	60	—	—	—	—
3	59	60	1(1)	—	—	—
4	58	60	3(3)	—	—	—
5	58	58	3(3)	1(1)	—	—
6	57	54	4(4)	3(4)	—	—
7	56	54	5(5)	6(7)	—	—
8	52	53	13(20)	7(9)	—	—
9	52	52	14(24)	11(21)	1(1)	1(1)
10	50	45	15(28)	15(29)	3(3)	2(2)
11	49	42	18(33)	15(29)	7(7)	2(2)
12	39	39	19(36)	17(31)	7(7)	5(5)
13	36	37	20(38)	21(35)	7(7)	5(5)
14	33	25	20(38)	26(51)	7(7)	7(7)

Each group was started with 60 mice.

115

TABLE 10. Benzo (a) Pyrene in Smoke Condensates*

Cigarette Type	Smoke Analysis					
	BaP			Phenol		
	$\mu g/g$	"tar"	$\mu g/cig$	$\mu g/g$	"tar"	$\mu g/cig$
Standard Tobacco Blend (30 cuts/inch)	1.05		29	3.46		96
Standard Tobacco Blend (Fine cut-50/inch)	1.22		30	3.65		88
Standard Tobacco Blend (Coarse cut-20/inch)	0.96		25	4.90		128
Standard Tobacco Blend + 8.3% $NaNO_3$	0.60		9.5	3.18		60
Standard Tobacco Blend + 5% $Cu(NO_3)_2$	0.68		20	2.86		86
100% Stems from Standard Tobacco Blend	1.29		16	4.68		58
100% Burley Tobacco (Low Nicotine)	0.94		24	2.35		60
100% Bright Tobacco	1.60		53	2.85		95
Hay (100%)	0.96		26	6.11		162
Spinach (100%)	0.69		11	5.00		79

* The cigarettes were all 85 mm long and were smoked under the same standard conditions. The experimental variations were, with the exception of the "hay" and "spinach-cigarettes" ±5% for phenol and ±8% for benzo (a) pyrene. The variation for the smoke of the non-tobacco cigarettes could not be estimated since the make-up of these cigarettes varied significantly.

lated to the activity of the test materials as a complete carcinogen, such a relationship does not exist for the promotion phase.[25]

DISCUSSION

Experimental tobacco carcinogenesis includes at least 3 phases—reduction in lung clearance, tumor initiation, and cocarcinogenesis including tumor promotion. In model experiments on mouse skin, we are mainly testing tumor initiation and tumor promotion. The published data strongly suggest that certain polynuclear aromatic hydrocarbons (PAH) represent the major tumor initiators in tobacco "tar." A significant reduction or increase of PAH results in a significant decrease or increase of the carcinogenicity of tobacco "tar" as measured on mouse skin. The majority of the PAH in the smoke are formed during the burning of tobacco. So far, several ways were tried to reduce the PAH. These include changing of the precursors for PAH, by tobacco selection, or by use of tobacco additives.[13, 24]

Our present knowledge of cocarcinogenic factors, in general, and tumor promoters in cigarette smoke condensate, in particular, is rather limited. In fact, the only known group of tumor promoters in tobacco smoke are the volatile phenols. Their reduction of up to 80% by selective filtration, however, did not lead to a reduction of tumor promoting activity. It was the design of this study to gain some knowledge of the biological aspects of tobacco promoting activity and of possible ways to reduce smoke components possessing such activity.

From the results of this study we draw the following conclusions:

1. Although "tar" from Bright tobacco exhibits a greater carcinogenicity than "tar" from Burley tobacco[23] both "tars" have comparable tumor promoting activity on mouse skin initiated with DMBA.

2. The degree of tobacco cut neither alters the tumor promoting activity of cigarette smoke condensate nor the complete tumorigenicity.[24]

3. Cigarette smoke condensate made from tobacco stems was found to have no tumor-promoting activity: in evaluating this finding it should be noted further that a "stem cigarette" delivers only 12.4 mg condensate and the standard cigarette 21.8 mg and that the stem cigarette is filled with 1.8 g tobacco compared to the standard cigarette with 1.09 g tobacco.

Darkis et al.[3, 4] have shown that in comparison with the laminar portions, all types of tobacco stems (midribs) have a low content of petroleum ether extractables, water soluble acids and nicotine; the latter factor is also reflected in the low nicotine content of the smoke and relatively small basic portion of the whole "tar" obtained from all "stem" cigarettes (4.2% compared to 10.0% for standard "tar"). Stems may have up to 25% of cellulose compared to up to 10% for the lamine portion of tobacco, and stems are estimated to be made up by up to 15% lignin.[17] Compared on a weight basis, however, stem "tar" is high in PAH as indicated with BaP and significantly higher in volatile phenols than the standard "tar."

116

The finding of decreased biological activity of "tars" from cigarettes made of tobacco stems or with stems added[24] is significant in that it parallels the decreased tumorigenicity observed of tobacco "tars" tested during the past 2 decades.[26] It is possible that the tumor-promoting activity of "tars" has decreased simultaneously in the same period, although comparable data are not available. Such reduction may be due at least in part to the greatly increased use of stems.

4. The tumor-promoting activity to mouse skin of spinach "tar" is similar to that of tobacco smoke condensate, while that of hay "tar" is lower. The activity of hay "tar" as a complete carcinogen is also significantly lower.

5. One of the most relevant findings of the present study is the similarity in tumor-promoting activity of equal doses of tobacco extract obtained with DMSO and cigarette smoke condensate. In an evaluation of these relative activities, we have to consider that the "tar" from the mainstream smoke amounts to only 3% of the cigarette weight burned and which is tested in the bioassay while extraction of tobacco yields 60% of its weight in test materials. Also DMSO may extract more of the tumor promoters from tobacco than "distill" into the smoke from the tobacco burned during puffing.

We suspect that some tobacco tumor promoters "distill" during smoking unaltered in basic structure into the mainstream smoke while others may be formed by pyrosynthesis. Nevertheless, we cannot exclude that the tobacco constituent(s) accounting for the promoting activity of the extract are different from those responsible for the activity in the smoke condensate. It is noteworthy that in a short-term test on mouse skin there is a marked hyperplastic effect with tobacco smoke condensate, whereas this effect is minimal with tobacco extracts.

The content of carcinogenic PAH in tobacco extracts is very low.[25] This supports the concept that these and related substances play an important role as tumor initiators.

CHEMICAL IDENTIFICATION OF TUMOR INITIATORS AND PROMOTERS

Previous studies by our group have demonstrated that tumor initiators are localized in a subfraction (BI) of the neutral portion of tobacco "tar." The carcinogenic PAH are concentrated in this fraction and their tumor initiating activity was found to be about 20 times greater than could be explained by the benzo(a)pyrene content. Therefore, we assume other tumor initiators of polynuclear aromatic hydrocarbon or similar structural type to be present in this fraction.[25, 26]

Evidence does not indicate such a clear delineation of a tumor promoting fraction in tobacco smoke condensate. Present data suggest that tumor promoters are present in several of the major fractions of tobacco "tar" as has been shown for the acidic and phenolic fractions (Table 1). The nicotine-free basic fraction, though lacking tumor-promoting activity, has significant hyperplastic activity on mouse skin.[25] In one experiment, in fact, papillomas were produced by such material, thus demonstrating a tumorigenic potential.[25] Pure phenol in a 5% concentration has been shown to promote tumors.[25] A reduction of phenol in tobacco smoke through the use of filters, however, does not alter the complete tumorigenic activity of "tar" obtained from such cigarettes. This infers that a selected reduction of volatile phenols will not reduce the tumor-promoting activity of such "tar." Similarly, negative results were shown when the volatile components of the smoke were reduced by using special filter material.

THEORETICAL CONSIDERATIONS

In evaluating cocarcinogenic properties of a given substance, different modes of action need to be considered. A particular substance may enhance the absorption of a carcinogen by facilitating its diffusion through the cellular membrane or by chemically affecting subcellular components. Another pathway is via the induction of chemical changes in cellular components which in turn stimulate the initiated but so far dormant tumor cell. In the present and most other experiments in tobacco carcinogenesis, the latter system has been the one primarily explored. In these studies, the mouse epidermis was first initiated with a subthreshold dose of a carcinogen and subsequently, tobacco "tar," tobacco extracts, or their various fractions were applied.

In this setting, we are testing tobacco products as promoters in the classical 2-step mechanism of carcinogenesis. Tobacco extract

117

and smoke contain substances capable of affecting chemical alterations of cellular components, which subsequently evoke the initiated tumor cells. Previous studies have indicated that certain tumor promoters adversely affect oxidative phosphorylation, and it has been shown that several tobacco smoke constituents can also accomplish this.[21] It may therefore be suggested that certain tobacco components act as tumor promoters by interference with mitochondrial respiration.

For tobacco products that possess complete carcinogenic properties, we also need to consider the total effect of the various complete carcinogens which are present in subthreshold concentrations. After 8–12 months when standard tobacco "tar" by itself can lead to tumor development, we can expect further development of tumors as a consequence of the effect of carcinogens (syncarcinogenesis) rather than from promoters. This may explain why after 12 months of application of standard "tar" more tumors are produced on initiated mouse skin than are observed with a high nitrate tobacco "tar" in which the PAH content is significantly lower.

Factors that may condition the immediate effect of a tumor initiator cannot be studied in the classical 2-step test. In future studies, the suspected cocarcinogen should be given concurrently with the initiator.

It is likely that on the basis of enhanced absorption some tobacco "tar" constituents can accelerate the carcinogenic effect of B(a)P. For instance, certain components present in fraction BI, which is the most active initiating fraction in tobacco "tar," may facilitate the absorption of known tobacco "tar" carcinogens.[13] This aspect of cocarcinogenesis needs to be explored further.

Another area that requires additional consideration is the apparent interrelation of noncarcinogenic aromatic hydrocarbons with carcinogenic PAH in skin carcinogenesis. We have shown that 4-ring hydrocarbons such as pyrene and fluoranthene, when given in a certain molecular ratio to B(a)P, increase the tumorigenicity of the carcinogen.[12] We should also mention the role of antagonists in carcinogenesis and cocarcinogenesis. Noncarcinogenic PAH have been shown capable of reducing the effect of structurally-related carcinogenic PAH.[5] Certain agents such as camphor can reduce the tumor promoting activity of phenol.[27] Compounds that delay absorption of carcinogens have been

shown to diminish the effects of B(a)P.[25] Homburger et al. have recently reviewed this aspect of carcinogenesis.[14]

It is apparent that cocarcinogenesis plays an important role in experimental tobacco carcinogenesis and that tumor initiators in tobacco "tar" play a decisive role at least in bioassays on mouse epithelium. A reduction of the tumor initiating fraction is accompanied by a reduction of the total carcinogenic activity of tobacco "tar." The present study indicates several approaches to how alteration of the various tobacco products could also lead to a reduction of their tumor-promoting properties.

SUMMARY AND CONCLUSIONS

1. Tobacco smoke condensate is an established tumor-promoter on mouse skin. When judged on a gram-to-gram basis, the tumor-promoting activity of a DMSO extract of Turkish tobacco is similar to that of the smoke condensate of a standard cigarette.

2. Tobacco type, the thickness of the tobacco cuts, nor the addition of nitrates influence the tumor-promoting activity of the resulting "tar."

3. "Tar" obtained from cigarettes made wholly of tobacco stems was found to have no tumor-promoting activity in the setting of this study.

4. Smoke condensate from hay cigarettes had low activity, both as a complete carcinogen and as a tumor promoter, while the smoke condensate of "spinach" cigarettes had a tumor-promoting activity similar to that of the standard cigarette.

5. The chemical nature and formation of tumor initiators and tumor promoters in tobacco smoke appear to be quite different. The main tumor initiators can be localized in a single "tar" subfraction, but the promoter appears to be spread over several of the major tobacco fractions. Consequently, identification of specific tumor promoters in tobacco smoke condensate will be more difficult.

6. Further research into the chemical identification of the major tumor promoting agents in tobacco smoke condensate and tobacco extracts must be a primary goal in experimental tobacco carcinogenesis.

REFERENCES

1. Bock, F. G., Moore, G. E., and Crouch, S. K.: Tumor-promoting activity of extracts of unburned tobacco. *Science* 145:831–833, 1964.

2. Clemo, G. R., and Miller, E. W.: Tumor promotion by the neutral fraction of cigarette smoke. *Brit. J. Cancer* 14:651–656, 1960.

3. Darkis, F. R. C., and Hackney, E. J.: Cigarette tobaccos. Chemical changes that occur during processing. *Ind. Eng. Chem.* 44:284–291, 1951.

4. ———, Baisden, L. A., Gross, P. M., and Wolf, F. A.: Flue-cured tobacco. Chemical composition of rib and blade tissue. *Ind. Eng. Chem.* 44:297–301, 1952.

5. Falk, H. L., Kotin, P., and Thompson, S. J.: Inhibition of carcinogenesis. *Arch. Environ. Health (Chicago)* 9:169–179, 1964.

6. Gellhorn, A.: Co-carcinogenic activity of cigarette tobacco tar. *Cancer Res.* 18:510–517, 1958.

7. Guérin, M.: Étude sur le pouvoir co-carcinogène du goudron de fumée de cigarette. *Bull. Assoc. Franc. Cancer* 48:365–376, 1961.

8. Gwynn, R. H., and Salaman, M. H.: Examination of an extract of cigarette tobacco and pure nicotine for carcinogenic and co-carcinogenic action on mouse skin. *Rept. Brit. Empire Cancer Campaign* 31:143, 1953.

9. ———: Studies on promotion of tumor development (co-carcinogenesis). *Report. Brit. Empire Cancer Campaign* 32:171–172, 1954.

10. ———, and Salaman, M. H.: Tests of products for tumor initiation and promotion in mouse skin. *Report. Brit. Empire Cancer Campaign* 34:193–194, 1956.

11. Hamer, D., and Woodhouse, D. L.: Biological tests for co-carcinogenic action of tar from cigarette smoke. *Brit. J. Cancer* 10:49–53, 1956.

12. Hoffmann, D., and Wynder, E. L.: Studies on gasoline engine exhaust. *J. Air. Pollut. Contr. Ass.* 13:323–327, 1963.

13. ———, and ———: Selective reduction of the tumorigenicity of tobacco smoke. Experimental approaches. *Nat. Cancer Inst. Monogr.* 28:157–172, 1968.

14. Homburger, F., Trieger, A., and Boger, E.: Experimental studies on the inhibition of carcinogenesis by cigarette smoke condensates and carcinogen-related substances. *Nat. Cancer Inst. Monogr.* 28:259–270, 1968.

15. Ranadive, K. J., Gothoskar, S. V., and Khavolkar, V. R.: Experimental studies on the etiology of cancer types specific to India. a) Oral cancer; b) Kangri cancer. *Acta Un. Int. Cancr.* 19:634–639, 1963.

16. Roe, F. J. C., Salaman, M. H., and Cohen, J.: Incomplete carcinogens in cigarette smoke condensate tumor-promotion by phenolic fraction. *Brit. J. Cancer* 13:623–633, 1959.

17. Samfield, M., and Christy, M. G.: The average of polymerization of cellulose in various tobacco types. Part II. Results. *Tobacco Sci.* 4:38–41, 1960.

18. Van Duuren, B. L., Sivak, A., and Langseth, L.: The tumor-promoting agents of tobacco leaf and tobacco smoke condensate. *J. Nat. Cancer Inst.* 37:519–526, 1966.

19. ———, ———, and ———: The tumor-promoting activity of tobacco leaf extract and whole cigarette tar. *Brit. J. Cancer* 21:460–463, 1967.

20. ———, ———, ———, Goldschmidt, B. M., and Segal, A.: Initiators and promoters in tobacco carcinogenesis. *Nat. Cancer Inst. Monogr.* 28:173–180, 1968.

21. Wilk, M., Bodenberger, A., and Wynder, E. L.: Unpublished data.

22. Wynder, E. L., and Hoffmann, D.: A study of tobacco carcinogenesis. VIII. The role of the acidic fractions as promoters. *Cancer* 14:1306–1315, 1961.

23. ———, and ———: Ein experimenteller Beitrag zur Tabakrauchkanzerogenese. *Deutsch. Med. Wschr.* 88:623–628, 1963.

24. ———, and ———: Reduction of tumorigenicity of cigarette smoke. An experimental approach. *JAMA* 192:88–94, 1965.

25. ———, and ———: Tobacco and Tobacco Smoke, Studies in experimental carcinogenesis. New York, N.Y. Academic Press, Inc., 1967.

26. ———, and ———: Experimental tobacco carcinogenesis. *Science* 162:862–871, 1968.

27. Wynder, E. L., and Lyons, M. J.: Unpublished data.

CHANGES IN MITOCHONDRIAL ULTRASTRUCTURE IN NICKEL SULFIDE-INDUCED RHABDOMYOSARCOMA

Parvathi K. Basrur, PhD, Anthony K. Sykes, and J. P. W. Gilman, DVM

INTRAMUSCULAR INJECTIONS OF NICKEL SALTS have been demonstrated to be capable of inducing tumors of striated muscle origin in rats.[10-14] Cellular changes similar to those noted during in vivo muscle tumorogenesis and a striking reduction in DNA synthesis were observed when cultures of embryonic muscle were exposed to nickel sulfide.[2] Although the striated muscle was consistently shown to be the tissue of preference for nickel compounds injected through various routes,[12] the primary targets of nickel in adult muscle and cultured embryonic muscle cells are not known. In an attempt to characterize the ultrastructural changes elicited by nickel sulfide, a group of rhabdomyosarcomas induced with nickel sulfide was examined and comparisons were made with adult muscle tissues exposed to this carcinogen for shorter durations. This report concerns changes in mitochondria which, besides being among the most important intracellular functional entities, appeared to be among the group of cell organelles to respond consistently to the presence of nickel in the cellular environment.

Material and Methods

The method of inducing rhabdomyosarcomas in rats has been described in detail elsewhere.[1, 11, 12] In the present experiments, powdered nickel sulfide, washed in several changes of phosphate buffered saline (PBS) was suspended in Ayercillin (300,000 I.U. penicillin G procaine per ml aqueous solution) for injection into the thigh muscles of 5- to 6-week-old Fischer rats. Each rat received 0.2 ml of the suspension containing 10 mg of nickel sulfide. Five rats of the same sex were housed in each of 4 metal cages and standard laboratory animal care was observed throughout the experiment.

In order to study the short-term effect of nickel sulfide, another group of 6 rats was injected with nickel sulfide as described above, with the exception that the amount of nickel in the suspension was reduced to 2.5 mg per rat. These rats were sacrificed at 24 and 48 hours after injection, and the tissues were processed for light and electron microscopic studies. The controls for this experiment included 2 groups of 10 rats each, of corresponding age. One group received injections with 0.2 ml PBS whereas the other group ,was injected with 0.2 ml Ayercillin alone.

Necrosis-free pieces of tumors and muscle tissues from areas free of particulate nickel was fixed in 3.5% glutaraldehyde,[23] for 3 hours, and the fixed tissues were stored for several days in 6.5% sucrose at 4 C prior to post-fixation in 1% osmium tetroxide for one hour. The fixatives and the sucrose solution were made up in 0.1M phosphate buffer at pH 7.4.[19] The fixed material was rinsed in distilled water, stained with a saturated aqueous solution of uranyl acetate for one hour, and dehydrated in graded series of alcohol and prophylene oxide before embedding in maraglas.[25]

All maraglas blocks were sectioned at 0.5 μ − 1.0 μ and stained with 0.5% toluidine blue in 1.0% borax,[18] to select areas of interest which were photographed under a Zeiss photomicroscope. Ultrathin sections of selected areas were cut on a Reichert OM-U2 ultramicrotome and stained with lead citrate,[31] for examination with a JEM-6A electron microscope.

Tissue samples from each tumor were also fixed in 10% neutral buffered formalin for histologic preparations and subsequent characterization of tumors.

RESULTS

In the group of rats receiving 10 mg of nickel sulfide, palpable tumors were apparent between 3 and 4 months after the injection. As in previous experiments, the control groups exhibited no tumors even after a year. Out of the 16 tumors in the 20 experimental animals, 11 were rhabdomyosarcomas (Figs. 1, 2) characterized by the presence of cross striated straps in both the primary tumors and their lung metastases. All tumors included in the present study were rhabdomyosarcomas in which the distribution of multinucleate strap cells and uninucleated dividing cells varied widely.

One of the consistent features of nickel sulfide-induced rhabdomyosarcomas concerned an alteration in the size and internal structure of mitochondria. There was a wide range in the size of mitochondria, with some being considerably more enlarged (Fig. 3). Some of the hypertrophied mitochondria exhibited an excessive build up of tubular units which appeared to have coalesced in groups or formed wavy or straight stacks (Fig. 4). The parallel stacks appeared to be continuous with the inner mitochondrial membrane and the cristae in several areas. Occasionally, circular profiles of the stack units were noted singly or in groups of 2 and 4 (Fig. 3). The diameter of these units appeared to be approximately half that of the "normal" cristae (Fig. 3, inset). The periphery of some of the cristae and that of the tubular units appeared to be consistently more electron dense (Figs. 3, 4). A multidirectional orientation of the stack units is indicated by the presence of circular and parallel aggregates side by side in some mitochondria (Fig. 5).

The internal structure of these mitochondria frequently showed varying degrees of degeneration characterized by the disruption and loss of cristae (Fig. 6). A more advanced state of alteration appeared in the form of total replacement of the inner constituents of mitochondria with 50 to 60 Å filaments (Fig. 7).

Intramitochondrial membrane thickening and coalescence of stack units were more apparent in tumor cells which appeared to be extremely dedifferentiated. A majority of such cells contained rough-surfaced endoplasmic reticulum and free ribosomes (Figs. 3–8). Aberrant mitochondria were also noted in mitotic cells (Fig. 8) and in myoblasts (Fig. 9) exhibiting distorted contractile elements.[9] Ultrastructurally altered mitochondria with extremely stretched parallel stacks were also noted in myoblasts appearing to be at earlier stages of contractile protein organization. The direction of the parallel stacks in some of these mitochondria appeared to follow the orientation of the myofilaments in the surrounding cytoplasm.

Normal muscles from untreated adult rats and from rats injected with PBS or Ayercillin did not exhibit any alterations in the internal structure of mitochondria. However, exposure to nickel sulfide for short periods seemed to elicit changes in mitochondria similar to those noted in the nickel sulfide-induced tumors. In muscle cells exposed to nickel sulfide for 24 or 48 hours, bead-like structures were noted in parallel rows in longitudinal sections and as peripheral aggregates in cross sections (Figs. 10–12). The accumulation of bead-like structures on the

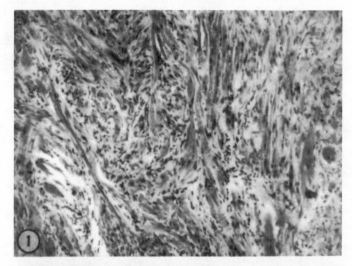

FIG. 1. A rhabdomyo-sarcoma from the site of nickel sulfide injection. Note the large number of muscle straps (H and E, ×150).

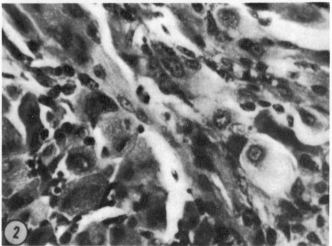

FIG. 2. A higher magnification of a typical rhabdomyosarcoma showing strap cells with distinct cross striations. Note the dividing cell close to a strap cell (H and E, ×500).

periphery was most striking in muscle cells exposed to nickel sulfide for 48 hours. Electron microscopic studies on these tissues confirmed the mitochondrial nature of the bead-like structures, and showed the alterations to include excessive proliferation and loss of orientation of cristae and accumulation of electron dense granules (Figs. 13, 14).

DISCUSSION

Aggregation of mitochondria: The electron microscopic studies on muscle tissue exposed to nickel sulfide for relatively short duration clearly indicated that a majority of mitochondria aggregating in longitudinal rows or in the periphery have altered internal structures. Whether the mitochondrial accumulation on the periphery of muscles is a passive phenomenon or a movement to facilitate the energy demand in the periphery where regenerative activities are envisaged is not known. The subsequent cellular changes leading to the dissociation of satellite cells and their assumed involvement in the reconstruction of the muscle tissue,[15, 22, 30] would seem

122

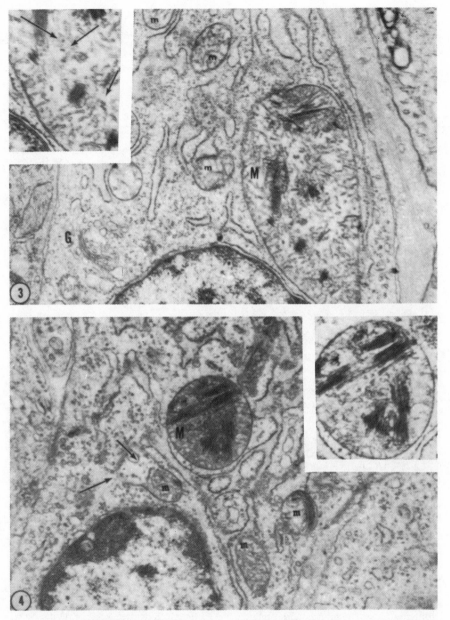

Fig. 3. The Golgi zone (G) of a cell from a nickel sulfide-induced rhabdomyosarcoma showing an altered mitochondrion (M) with aggregates of parallel tubules and several smaller mitochondria (m), ×27,500. Inset shows part of the altered mitochondrion (M) in which cross sections of 2 types of tubular units can be detected. The arrows indicate the smaller tubules occurring singly or in groups of 2 or 4 (×35,000).

Fig.4. Another rhabdomyosarcoma cell showing an abberant mitochondrion (M) with parallel stacks which are continuous with the cristae. Note the smaller mitochondria (m) which show focal disruption of the surface membranes (arrows) and continuity with the cisternae of the rough endoplasmic reticulum (×22,000). Inset shows tubular units in parallel stacks. All the stacks were seldom noted in focus. The upper 2 stacks of tubular units are in focus (×35,000).

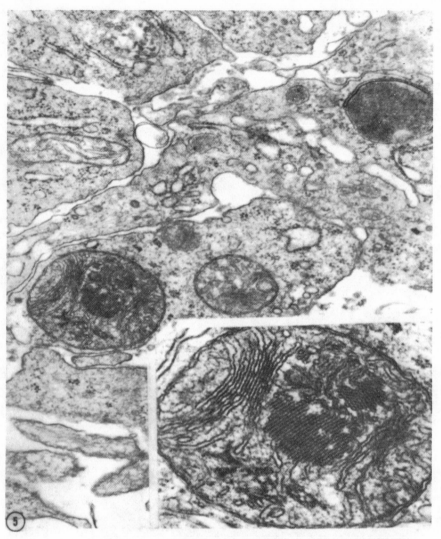

Fig. 5. Mitochondria from the cytoplasmic extensions of tumor cells. Note the lysosome-like bodies with and without a membrane and the mitochondria exhibiting internal alterations (×17,000). Inset shows one of the mitochondria at higher magnification. The thickened mitochondrial membranes appearing to be continuous with the inner membrane and electron dense areas probably representing damaged cristae may be noted (×35,000).

to indicate that the mitochondrial migration to the periphery is directed by the local energy requirement. Aggregation of mitochondria in the periphery of muscle cells has been reported in chicks, rats, and rabbits subjected to vitamin E deficiency,[4, 30] in rat muscle cells exposed to severe cold,[22] and in human rhabdomyosarcoma cells in the process of redifferentiation.[9] Such mitochondrial aggregates may be indicative of a nonspecific response of mus-

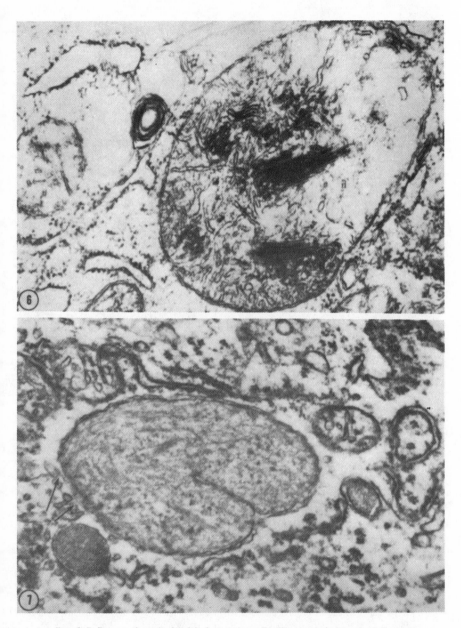

Figs. 6, 7. Degenerating mitochondria from tumor cells. The accumulations of tubular units and the focal dissolution of intramitochondrial architecture are evident in the mitochondrion in Fig. 7. Total replacement of mitochondrial interior with thin 50 to 60 Å filaments (arrows) is noticeable in Fig. 8. Note the lysosomes near the degenerating mitochondria (Fig. 7). (Fig. 6: ×49,000; Fig. 7: ×45,000)

125

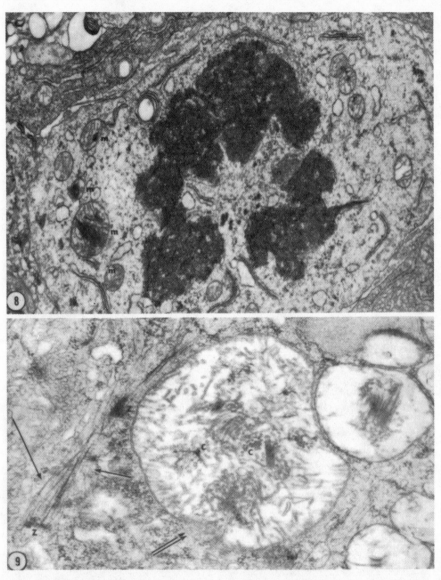

Fig. 8. A mitotic cell from a rhabdomyosarcoma showing several mitochondria (m) with dark parallel stacks of tubules. A "persistant nucleolus" (n) attached to one of the metaphase chromosomes and numerous paired membranes characteristic of the mitotic cells in these tumors may be noted (×18,000).

Fig. 9. A myoblast exhibiting several abnormal mitochondria. Note the circular profiles of cristae with thick membranes (C) within the large mitochondrion in the center and the thick and thin filaments (arrows) and the Z line materials (Z) in the cytoplasm indicating redifferentiation in a striated muscle cell derivative. Myofilaments can be noted extruding into the mitochondrion (double arrow), ×27,500.

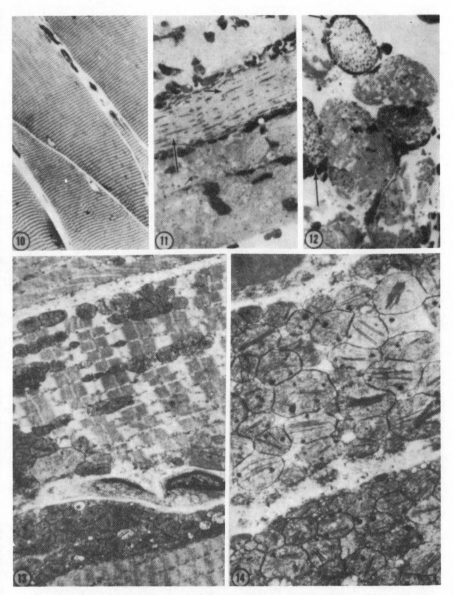

Figs. 10–12. Thin sections of maraglas embedded adult rat muscle exposed to 2.5 mg nickel sulfide (Toluidine blue-borax stain, ×500). Fig. 10. Normal skeletal muscle from the thigh of an adult Fischer rat. Fig. 11. Rat muscle cells exposed to nickel sulfide for 24 hours. Note the prominent mitochondria in parallel rows (arrows) resembling strings of beads. Fig. 12. Cross sections of muscle cells exposed to nickel sulfide for 48 hours, showing accumulation of mitochondria on the periphery (arrows).

Figs. 13, 14. Electron micrographs of adult muscle exposed to 2.5 mg of nickel sulfide for 24 hours. Fig. 13. Adult muscle exposed to 2.5 mg of nickel sulfide for 24 hours. Accumulation of mitochondria in parallel rows and in the periphery of muscle cells showing damaged contractile elements (×8,500). Fig. 14. Adult muscle exposed to 2.5 mg of nickel sulfide for 48 hours. Periphery of muscle cells showing accumulation of electron dense aggregates and the occurrence of parallel stacks in mitochondria (×15,000).

127

cle cells to insults of various kinds. However, in all instances involving a physical trauma or the depletion of such naturally occurring antioxidents as vitamin E,[28, 30] regeneration appeared to have been the pattern while the nickel sulfide-induced changes have consistently led to the development of rhabdomyosarcomas.

Mitochondrial substructure: A striking feature of the skeletal muscle exposed to suboptimal amounts of nickel sulfide was the change in the internal structure of mitochondria simulating that noted in nickel-induced rhabdomyosarcomas. Although alterations in the internal structure of mitochondria have been reported in human rhabdomyomas,[5, 6, 9] and under environmental conditions influenced by acid pH,[3] estrogenic hormones,[8] and vitamin E deficiency,[4, 30] the changes noted in the present instance would seem to be unique in that every mitochondrion in muscles exposed to nickel sulfide for short periods and a good proportion of those present in the tumor cells were altered in their ultrastructural architecture in a characteristic manner. Also, in the present study, one of the initial cytologic changes noted appeared to be the swelling of mitochondria and the extreme proliferation of cristae which probably preceded their coalescence to form "stacks." In many instances, the parallel stacks were clearly detectable as continuous with the cristae which in cross sections appeared to be relatively more thickened than those of some of the apparently unaffected muscle mitochondria.

The internal alterations leading to the replacement of cristae with 50 to 60 Å filaments in rhabdomyosarcoma cells would appear to be mediated by the lytic organelles which have frequently been noted in the vicinity of affected mitochondria (Figs. 5, 7). Novikoff and Essner,[20] had suggested that the degenerating mitochondria may show the presence of acid phosphatase and that some of these may give rise to vacuoles. It is conceivable that the "altered" mitochondria represent stages in the focal renewal while the damaged mitochondria are being digested. A tendency for vacuole formation is evident in some mitochondria (Fig. 9) while others indicate replacement of the internal structure with irregular electron dense material (Fig. 5) or filamentous structures. It is possible that the filaments represent actin which is similar in thickness (50–60 Å) and has been

chemically identified within some mitochondria. These actin-like filaments noted in "altered" mitochondria may have originated as extra mitochondrial filaments similar to those reported in myoblasts and in various other cell types.[16] An indication of myofilament intrusion into altered mitochondria was apparent at least in some instances (Fig. 9) in the present study.

Possible physiologic significance of mitochondrial alterations: The accumulation of electron dense granules in mitochondria and the alteration of mitochondrial structure in muscle exposed to nickel sulfide may be indicative of a direct effect of nickel on mitochondrial membranes, which are known to be sensitive to cations. Peachey,[24] had observed accumulation of divalent cations like calcium, strontium, and barium in "granules" localized in mitochondrial matrix when isolated mitochondria or whole cells were bathed in medium containing these metals. It is conceivable that nickel, like these cations, replaces the metal ions already present in the intramitochondrial granules which are purportedly involved in the regulation of the internal ionic environment. It has been demonstrated that damage to the cell with such agents as irradiation will result in the uptake of metals including nickel, by mitochondrion.[8] If the cellular trauma from the implanted nickel sulfide was causally related to the change in mitochondrial structure, the initial dissolution of cross striations from the adult muscle close to the implants (Figs. 13, 14) can be considered concomitant of mitochondrial malfunctions, since muscle cells require mitochondria-generated ATP for the maintenance of normal structure and function of the various contractile elements.

Heath and Webb,[14] had observed some accumulation of tumor-inducing metals, including nickel, in the mitochondrial fractions although the nuclear fractions of tissues from the implantation site had exhibited the greatest concentration of inducing metals. It is possible that the nickel incorporated in the mitochondria specifically affects the sulfhydryl proteins or the −SH enzymes such as succinic dehydrogenase which is distributed mainly in mitochondria.[17] In a previous investigation, we had demonstrated that nickel has an effect on the −SH proteins of the mitotic spindle.[27] Recently Saito and Ogawa,[24] reported mitochondrial aberrations in rat hepatic parenchymal cells. These workers have postulated that the aberration may be associated with the swelling-contraction mechanisms associated with respiration. The aberrant mitochondria noted in hepatic cells,[24, 26] and in muscle cells exposed to nickel, may represent a hypofunctional phase of mitochondria in terms of oxidative respiration. Histochemical studies on precancerous tissues and nickel sulfide-induced tumors have shown that there was a drop in succinic dehydrogenase activity in the former, although in well-differentiated rhabdomyosarcomas this enzyme was relatively more elevated than in tumors of nonmuscle origin.[29] Spycher and Rüttner[26] have noted ultrastructurally altered mitochondria similar to those seen in the present investigation in a variety of liver diseases in humans where altered metabolic function of the hepatic cells have been demonstrated. If such a functional alteration is induced by nickel in muscle mitochondria, it would appear that the altered state is compatible with cell reproduction since they are present in a majority of cells contributing to to the growth of rhabdomyosarcoma. Their presence in apparently degenerative muscle cells and in myoblasts exhibiting abnormal organization of the contractile proteins seems to indicate that the altered mitochondria interfere with muscle differentiation. It is conceivable that the enlarged mitochondria noted in tumors are derivatives of the original mitochondria of the adult muscle which have been structurally altered in response to the nickel sulfide in the cellular environment. Smaller mitochondria exhibiting normal morphology in these tumor cells are probably derived from the unaffected mitochondrial populations during repeated cell division.

The association of abnormal mitochondria with the other organelles in the cells is worthy of note. They are generally more abundant in the Golgi zone and in the vicinity of microbodies and multivesicular bodies. In a majority of instances the endoplasmic reticulum surrounding these mitochondria seemed to be active in that their cisternae, filled with amorphous substances, were continuous with the enlarged mitochondria. Saito and Ogawa,[24] also have reported an intimate topographic relationship of the aberrant mitochondria with the Golgi zone and the rough-surfaced endoplasmic reticulum. Their association with the rough-surfaced endoplasmic reticulum seems to suggest a metabolic interrelation. The change in mitochondria may be influenced by the synthetic activity of the cells which are undergoing dedifferentiation from highly specialized normal muscle cells to mononucleated cells capable of repeated cell division within an environment altered by nickel sulfide.

REFERENCES

1. Basrur, P. K., and Gilman, J. P. W.: The behaviour of two cell strains derived from rat rhabdomyosarcomas. *J. Nat. Cancer Inst.* 30:163–201, 1963.

2. ———, and Gilman, J. P. W.: Morphologic and synthetic response of normal and tumor muscle cultures to nickel sulfide. *Cancer Res.* 27:1168–1177, 1967.

3. Cereijo-Santalo, R.: Mitochondrial swelling at acid pH. *Canad. J. Biochem.* 44:695–706, 1966.

4. Cheville, N. F.: The pathology of vitamin E deficiency in the chick. *Path. Vet. (Basel)* 3:208–225, 1966.

5. Cornog, J. L., Jr., and Gonatas, N. K.: Ultrastructure of rhabdomyoma. *J. Ultrastruct. Res.* 20:433–450, 1967.

6. Czernobilsky, B., Cornog, J. L., and Enterline, H. T.: Rhabdomyoma. Report of case with ultrastructural and histochemical studies. *Amer. J. Clin. Path.* 49:782–789, 1968.

7. Decker, W. J.: The influence of lethal X-irradiation on trace metal uptake by the mitochondrion. *Experientia* 24:448–449, 1968.

8. Dietrich, L. S., Friedland, J. J., and Cefalu, R. C.: Mitochondrial swelling produced by compounds exhibiting estrogenic activity. *Proc. Soc. Exp. Biol. Med.* 107:168–170, 1961.

9. Freeman, A. I., and Johnson, W. W.: A comparative study of childhood rhabdomyosarcoma and virus-induced rhabdomyosarcoma in mice. *Cancer Res.* 28:1490–1500, 1968.

10. Gilman, J. P. W.: I. Observations on the carcinogenicity of a refinery dust, cobalt oxide, and colloidal thorium dioxide. *Cancer Res.* 22:152–157, 1962.

11. ———: Muscle tumorigenesis. Plse. *6th Canad. Cancer Conf.* 209–223, 1965.

12. ———, and Ruckerbauer, G. M.: Metal carcinogenesis II. A study on the carcinogenic activity of cobalt, copper, iron and nickel compounds. *Cancer Res.* 22:158–162, 1962.

13. Heath, J. C., and Daniel, M. R.: The production of malignant tumors by nickel in the rat. *Brit. J. Cancer* 18:261–264, 1964.

14. ———, and Webb, M.: Content and intracellular distribution of the inducing metal in the primary rhabdomyosarcomata induced in rat by cobalt, nickel and cadmium. *Brit. J. Cancer* 21:768–778, 1967.

15. Howes, E. L., Jr., Price, H. M., and Blumberg, M. M.: The effects of a diet producing lipochrome pigment (ceroid) on the ultrastructure of skeletal muscle in the rat. *Amer. J. Path.* 45:599–630, 1964.

16. Ishikawa, H., Bischoff, R., and Holtzer, H.: Mitosis and intermediate sized filaments in developing skeletal muscle. *J. Cell. Biol.* 38:538–552, 1968.

17. Lehninger, A. L.: The Mitochondrion. Molecular Basis of Structure and Function. New York, W. A. Benjamin Inc., 1964.

18. Mercer, E. H.: A scheme for section staining in electron microscopy. *J. Roy. Micr. Soc.* 81:179–186, 1963.

19. Millonig, G.: Further observations on a phosphate buffer of osmium solution in fixation. *In* Electron Microscopy. Fifth Intern. Congress Philadelphia, vol. 2. New York, Academic Press, 1962; p. 8.

20. Novikoff, A. B., and Essner, E.: Cytolysomes and mitochondrial degeneration. *J. Cell Biol.* 15:140–146, 1962.

21. Peachey, L. D.: Electron microscopic observations on the accumulation of divalent cations in intramitochondrial granules. *J. Cell Biol.* 20:95–109, 1964.

22. Price, H. M., Howes, E. L., and Blumberg, J. M.: Ultrastructural alterations in skeletal muscle injured by cold. II. Cells of the sarcolemmal tubes: observations on discontinuous regeneration and myofibril formation. *Lab. Invest.* 13:1279–1302, 1964.

23. Sabatini, D. D., Bensch, K., and Barrnett, R. J.: Cytochemistry and electron microscopy. The preservation of cellular ultrastructure and enzymatic activity by aldehyde fixation. *J. Cell Biol.* 17:19–58, 1963.

24. Saito, T., and Ogawa, K.: Aberrant mitochondria with longitudinal cristae observed in the normal rat hepatic parenchymal cells. *Okajima. Folia Anat. Jap.* 44:357–363, 1968.

25. Spurlock, B. O., Kattine, V. C., and Freeman, J. A.: Technical modification in maraglas embedding. *J. Cell Biol.* 17:203–207, 1963.

26. Spycher, M. A., and Rüttner, J. R.: Kristalloide Einschlüsse in menschlichen Lebermitochondrien. *Virchow. Arch. Zellpath.* 1:211–221, 1968.

27. Swierenga, S. H. H., and Basrur, P. K.: Effects of nickel sulfide on cultured muscle cells. *Lab. Invest.* 19:663–674, 1968.

28. Tappel, A. L.: Vitamin E as the biological lipid antioxidant. *Vitamins Hormones* 20:493–510, 1962.

29. Tsai, K.: Enzyme histochemical studies on muscle tumorigenesis and on nickel induced rhabdomyosarcomas. M.Sc. Thesis, University of Guelph, April 1966.

30. Van Vleet, J. F., Hall, B. V., and Simon, J.: Vitamin E deficiency: a sequential study by means of light and electron microscopy of alterations occuring in regeneration of skeletal muscle of affected weanling rabbits. *Amer. J. Path.* 51:815–830, 1967.

31. Venable, J. H., and Coggeshall, R.: A simplified lead citrate stain for use in electron microscopy. *J. Cell Biol.* 25:407–408, 1965.

PHYSIOLOGICAL GENETICS OF MELANOTIC TUMORS IN *DROSOPHILA MELANOGASTER*. VI. THE TUMORIGENIC EFFECTS OF JUVENILE HORMONE-LIKE SUBSTANCES

PETER J. BRYANT AND JAMES H. SANG

GENETICALLY determined melanotic tumors of Drosophila arise by the aggregation and subsequent melanisation of blood cells during larval life. They persist into the adult stage as apparently inert masses which either float freely in the haemolymph, or are associated with the fat body. The blood cells chiefly involved in tumorigenesis are the lamellocytes ("spindle cells"), which are derived by a transformation from the predominant blood cells, the plasmatocytes (OFTEDAL 1953; RIZKI 1960; SANG and BURNET 1963). RIZKI (1960) found that this transformation occurs in wild-type strains at about the time of metamorphosis, and he produced evidence to show that the transformation is under hormonal control. He showed that melanotic tumor strains are characterized by a premature blood cell transformation, and suggested that the metabolic defect underlying tumorigenesis may be in the hormonal system which controls metamorphosis. Support for this hypothesis comes from the finding that, in tumorous strains, tumor frequency can be altered by interfering with hormonal function by means of ligature (BURDETTE 1954; RIZKI 1960; see also SANG and BURNET 1963).

Any mutation involving the endocrine system of an insect would be extremely useful for the analysis of hormonal mechanisms, so it is important to explore the relationship between endocrine events and tumorigenesis in order to test RIZKI's hypothesis, and to delineate the type of defect, if one exists, in melanotic tumor strains. Several materials with hormonal activity for insects have recently become available, thus allowing a new approach to the problem, involving direct administration of these materials to the growing larvae as suggested by BURNET and SANG (1964b). The compounds we have examined are mimics of the juvenile hormone, and although there have been few reports of juvenile hormone effects on the higher Diptera (BRYANT and SANG 1968; SRIVASTAVA and GILBERT 1969), we have been able to show that many of these materials are very active in modifying the expression of melanotic tumor genes.

MATERIALS AND METHODS

The melanotic tumor gene with which we have been chiefly concerned is at locus 83.9 on the second chromosome (GLASS 1954) and is carried by the strain $tu\ bw;+^{su-tu}$. The tumor penetrance in this strain is approximately 90% when larvae are grown aseptically on defined medium under our conditions. The following tumor strains were also used in some experiments: $tu55g$ (JACOBS, BOWMAN and WALLISER 1958); tu^K (SANG and BURNET 1963); and $tu^W rc$ (RIZKI 1960). Larvae were raised aseptically, following the procedure of SANG (1956). The constitution of the defined medium was based on medium C of this author, but differed from it in that (i) sucrose was used instead of fructose, to minimize the "browning" reaction with amino acids during autoclaving; (ii) the medium contained magnesium (as sulphate), a requirement demonstrated by SANG (1956) which is not satisfied by the magnesium content of Oxoid No. 3 agar (SANG and BURNET 1967); (iii) K_2HPO_4 replaced Na_2HPO_4, to give a more optimal sodium/potassium ratio (BRYANT 1967). 5 ml or 2 ml of medium was dispensed into 15×2.5 cm test tubes, which were stoppered, autoclaved and cooled. Eggs were collected and sterilised following SANG's (1956) method. They were dechorionated with saturated calcium hypochlorite solution, and sterilised by rinsing in 0.1% cetyl dimethyl benzyl ammonium chloride solution (a quaternary ammonium detergent), using for the latter purpose a reversing pump of the type described by SANG (1956). Sterile eggs were plated onto agar in Petri dishes and incubated at 25°C. At about 20 hrs after egg collection, the hatched larvae were transferred, using paper spoons under sterile conditions, into tubes containing defined medium. A standard number of 40 larvae was used for each culture, with five replicate cultures for each test. Cultures were raised at 25°C in a humid incubator and any which became infected were discarded. Dosages were measured in millimoles per litre (mM) and plotted on logarithmic scales; the maximum concentration tested was usually 20mM or less. Emerged adults were counted twice daily, and the average time of development to adult was computed for each test.

The manifestation of melanotic tumor genes has usually been quantified by measuring tumor penetrance; that is, the proportion of tumorous flies in the population (SANG and BURNET 1963; BURNET and SANG 1964a, 1964b; GLASS 1957). However, this method is useful only for populations in which the gene shows incomplete penetrance, and near the upper end of the penetrance scale, measurements become inaccurate unless very large populations are used. Many of the populations involved in the experiments to be described had very high tumor penetrance, and for this reason the number of tumors present in each adult fly was counted. SANG's (1966) fructose clearing method was used, since this renders tumors visible without dissection of the flies. The mean number of tumors per fly was used as the parameter of tumor gene manifestation, and this will be referred to as tumor expression.

RESULTS

Effects of hormonally active materials on tumor expression: Several juvenile hormone mimics, and some related compounds, were tested for their effects on tumor expression in the melanotic tumor strain, $tu\ bw;+^{su\text{-}tu}$, and the results of these experiments are presented in Figures 1–15. Developmental time to adult was also measured, as an indicator of non-specific effects on development, but these results will not be presented in detail. At concentrations which were sufficient to modify tumor expression, most of the materials tested caused some delay in development, but the extent of this delay was not related to the juvenile hormone activity of the material concerned. None of the materials was found to induce supernumerary larval moults, as some of them do in certain other insects (LEVINSON 1966; WIGGLESWORTH 1963).

It was found convenient to feed these compounds directly to the larvae, rather than to attempt to inject them, so they were mixed with the defined medium before autoclaving. Since most of the materials in question were not water-soluble, they probably existed in the medium as a solution in globules of lecithin, which is the dietary source of fat. Larvae were in continuous contact with the food; thus both epidermal and alimentary cells were directly exposed to the chemicals. That

132

this is an effective means of administration is shown by the fact that a farnesoate derivative, applied in this way, causes results reminiscent of true juvenile hormone effects in other insects (BRYANT and SANG 1968).

Farnesol, farnesal, farnesene, nerolidol, phytol, isophytol: Farnesol is a triterpene primary alcohol, while farnesal is the corresponding aldehyde, farnesene the corresponding alkene, and nerolidol the 3-hydroxy isomer. Phytol differs from farnesol in its larger size and greater degree of saturation, and isophytol is the 3-hydroxy isomer of phytol. The relative juvenile hormone activities of these compounds are not always consistent, as reported by different authors using various test species. However the activities of farnesol, farnesal, nerolidol and phytol are usually of the same order of magnitude, although farnesal is consistently more active than farnesol, which is usually more active than nerolidol (KARLSON 1963; SCHMIALEK 1963; SCHNEIDERMAN et al. 1965). Isophytol, apparently, has no juvenile hormone activity (SCHNEIDERMAN and GILBERT 1964), and that of farnesene is extremely low (SCHNEIDERMAN et al. 1965).

These materials were tested over extensive dose ranges, and the results are presented in Figures 1–5. They all lower tumor expression quite markedly when the concentration is 2.5 mM or above, with the exception of farnesene which has no effect on tumor expression at concentrations up to 12mM. Since the dose response curves for these effects are rarely straight lines, and since the shape of the curve varies between treatments, it is not possible to express relative activities of the compounds by simple numbers, as has been found possible with their juvenile hormone activities. However, the data show that the order of decreasing tumor-suppressing activity is farnesol>nerolidol>isophytol>phytol>farnesal>farnesene. This order of activities does not correspond with the order of juvenile hormone activities as reported by any of the authors mentioned above. For example, farnesal is much more active than nerolidol or phytol, when measured using Tenebrio (SCHMIALEK 1963) and is also more active than farnesol when measured using Galleria (SCHNEIDERMAN and GILBERT 1964). Hence a comparison of the relative activities of these materials indicates that their tumor-suppressing properties are not correlated with, and therefore are probably not a result of their juvenile hormone potencies.

Farnesyl ethers and farnesyl diethylamine: Farnesyl methyl ether and farnesyl diethylamine have repeatedly been found to show roughly equal juvenile hormone activity, at least ten times as great as that of farnesol (BOWERS and THOMPSON 1963; KARLSON 1963; ROMAŇUK, SLÁMA and ŠORM 1967; SCHMIALEK 1963; SCHNEIDERMAN et al. 1965; WIGGLESWORTH 1963). Their effects on tumor expression in *tu bw*;+$^{su-tu}$, however, are completely different. Farnesyl methyl ether causes a significant elevation of tumor expression when the concentration is 0.5mM or above (Figure 6), and this compound can cause a much greater effect than is shown in the response curve when fed at a concentration of 4mM, especially in the *tu55g* strain, as will be shown later. Farnesyl diethylamine, on the other hand, causes a marked decrease in tumor expression when fed at 0.5mM (Figure 7), and probably would do so at a lower concentration. Thus it is more active in this respect than farnesol. This complete difference in activity between

133

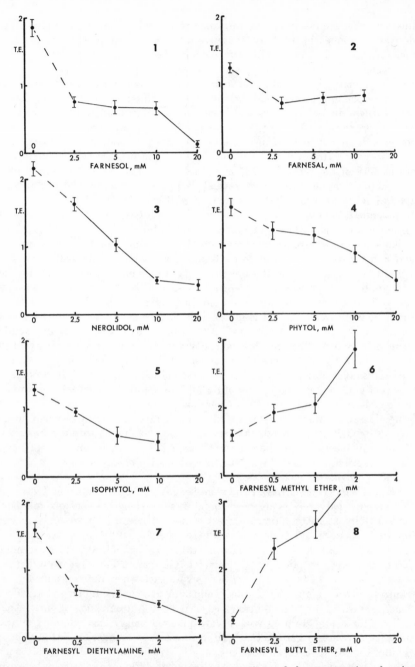

FIGURES 1–15.—The relation between tumor expression and the concentration of various materials in the larval medium, for the *tu bw;+su-tu* strain. Tumor expression (T.E.) is the average number of tumors developed per fly, and the vertical bars represent ± the standard

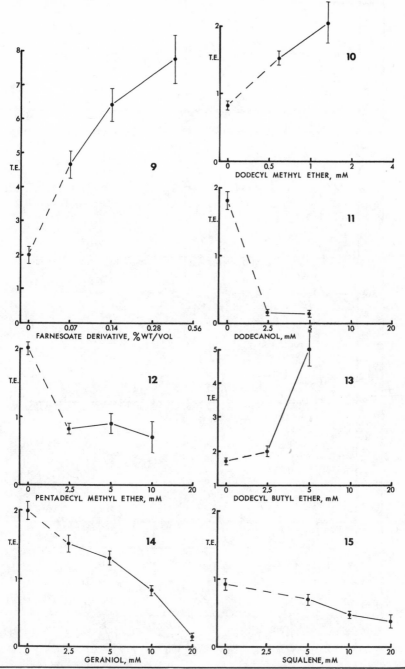

error of this parameter. Dosages are millimolar concentrations except for Figure 9 where the dose is measured as % wt./vol.

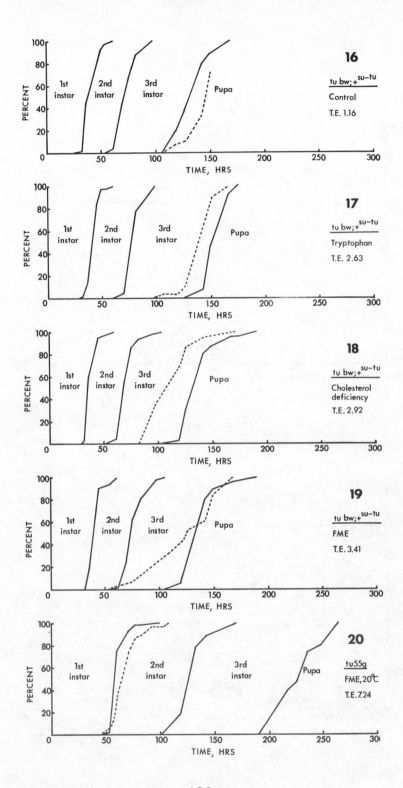

136

the two compounds must indicate that their site of action for effects on tumors is remarkably specific, and that this specificity is different from that of their juvenile hormone effects in other insects. This conclusion is reinforced by the finding that farnesyl butyl ether has tumorigenic activity as great as that of the methyl ether (Figure 8) although its juvenile hormone effects are much weaker, at least in Galleria (SCHMIALEK 1963; SCHNEIDERMAN et al. 1965).

Farnesoate derivative: LAW, YUAN and WILLIAMS (1966) synthesized a material from farnesoic acid by treatment with ethanolic HCl, and this substance was found to have extremely high juvenile hormone activity, although it was not a pure compound. It is the only juvenile hormone mimic which has been reported as showing effects in Diptera. It causes arrest of metamorphosis at various times depending on the dose, in mosquitoes and in Drosophila, and it also prevents the ontogenetic rotation of the male genitalia in these organisms (BRYANT and SANG 1968; SPIELMAN and SKAFF 1967). A sample of this material was tested on the $tu\ bw; +^{su-tu}$ strain at three levels: 0.07%, 0.14% and 0.35% wt./vol. At these concentrations, this material causes arrest of metamorphosis, so that tumors were scored in pupae for this experiment. Figure 9 shows that the arrested pupae had an extremely high tumor expression, the value being 7.73 tumors per fly at the maximum concentration tested, which is the highest yet recorded for this strain. Hence the most potent juvenile hormone mimic available to us is the most potent agent we have found for increasing tumor expression in $tu\ bw; +^{su-tu}$.

Straight-chain alcohols and ethers: SCHNEIDERMAN et al. (1965) showed that several long chain ethers had juvenile hormone activity in the Galleria wax test. The most active was dodecyl methyl ether, and decyl, undecyl, tridecyl and tetradecyl methyl ethers showed lower activity although the corresponding alcohols were completely inactive. Dodecyl ethyl ether had less activity than the methyl ether, and the butyl ether was almost inactive, indicating that the critical feature of the molecule was probably its size. Dodecyl methyl ether showed high activity in Tenebrio (BOWERS and THOMPSON, 1963), and dodecanol was also active in this species.

Most of these compounds have been tested for their effects on tumorigenesis in the $tu\ bw; +^{su-tu}$ strain, and the results are presented in Figures 10–13. Dodecyl

---

FIGURES 16–20.—Patterns of larval development. Solid lines represent the percentage of visible animals in the next instar at various times. Dotted lines represent the percentage of visible larvae with macroscopically visible melanotic tumors.

Figure 16. $tu\ bw; +^{su-tu}$ strain, grown on control medium.
Figure 17. $tu\ bw; +^{su-tu}$ strain, grown on medium containing 50mM L-tryptophan.
Figure 18. $tu\ bw; +^{su-tu}$ strain, grown on medium containing 0.001% cholesterol (control medium contains 0.03%).
Figure 19. $tu\ bw; +^{su-tu}$ strain, grown on medium containing 4mM farnesyl methyl ether.
Figure 20. $tu55g$ strain, grown at 20°C on medium containing 6mM farnesyl methyl ether.
The results are based on sample sizes of 50–170 animals. The tumor expressions attained by the populations are indicated in the figures.

137

methyl ether and dodecanol affect the tumor system in opposite directions, just as do farnesyl methyl ether and farnesol. Dodecyl methyl ether is about as active as farnesyl methyl ether in increasing tumor expression, while dodecanol is even more active than farnesol in decreasing it. When the length of the longer chain of the ether is increased, there is a falling off of tumorigenic activity, just as there is a decrease of juvenile hormone activity; tridecyl and tetradecyl methyl ethers (up to 10mM) have no detectable effect on tumor expression, and pentadecyl methyl ether causes a lowering of tumor expression (Figure 12). However, an increase in the length of the short chain of the ether, although it results in loss of juvenile hormone activity (SCHNEIDERMAN et al. 1965), does not abolish tumorigenic activity, as is shown by the potent effect of dodecyl butyl ether (Figure 13). An exactly similar situation was noted above in the case of the farnesyl ethers.

Geraniol, linalool, squalene: Geraniol, farnesol, linalool and squalene are of interest in that they are related to intermediates in the biosynthesis of cholesterol in vertebrate tissues (BLOCH 1965). Insects do not synthesize cholesterol (CLAYTON 1964), but as juvenile hormone is structurally related to the terpenes, it may be synthesized via the cholesterol pathway. Geraniol and its 3-hydroxy isomer, linalool, have shown low juvenile hormone activity in some tests, and where both have been tested, linalool has shown greater activity than geraniol (GILBERT and SCHNEIDERMAN 1964; SCHMIALEK 1963). Geraniol (Figure 14) reduces tumor expression in the tu $bw;+^{su-tu}$ strain, its effect being roughly comparable to that of phytol (Figure 4), but linalool has absolutely no effect on tumor expression, in spite of causing a retardation of development similar to that of geraniol. Hence the 1-3 isomerisation of geraniol results in loss of tumor-suppressing activity, but does not cause loss of juvenile hormone activity. It is surprising, therefore, that the same isomerisation of farnesol (to nerolidol) results in loss of neither activity (Figures 1 and 3), whereas a similar change in the phytol molecule (to isophytol) results in loss of juvenile hormone activity but has little effect on tumor-suppressing properties (Figures 4 and 5). Squalene also reduces tumor expression, its effectiveness being similar to that of phytol (Figure 15).

The time course of tumor formation: The above results add substantially to the already impressive array of environmental treatments which have been shown to be capable of influencing quantitatively the development of melanotic tumors (SANG and BURNET 1967). However, the fact that particular treatments can influence tumor penetrance or expression tells us little of the mechanism of these effects, and a search for qualitative differences in responses to various treatments seems to be required. We have begun such a study by examining the time of tumor formation under various environmental and genetic circumstances, and we have found that there are indeed marked variations in the time when tumors appear.

Environmental influences on the time of tumor formation: Figures 16–19 show the time of appearance of macroscopically visible melanotic tumors in the tu $bw;$ $+^{su-tu}$ strain grown under four different dietary conditions: control; supplementary tryptophan (50mM); cholesterol deficiency (0.001%); and farnesyl methyl ether (FME), (4mM). The instar changes in these populations are plotted on the figures, and the tumor expression in the adults is also indicated.

In the control series (Figure 16), visible melanized tumors do not appear until late in the third larval instar, which is the usual time of tumor formation in strains carrying tu bw (BURNET and SANG 1964b) or other melanotic tumor genes (GUÉLÉLOVITCH 1958; JACOBS et al. 1958; OFTEDAL 1953; RIZKI 1960; SANG and BURNET 1963). However when tumor expression is increased by means of supplementary tryptophan or by cholesterol deficiency (Figures 17 and 18), tumors appear somewhat earlier during the third instar, and the more potent tumorigenic treatment (cholesterol deficiency) causes more precocious tumor formation. With the still more potent tumorigenic agent, FME, tumors appear even earlier than with cholesterol deficiency (Figure 19); in fact, out of the sample of 141 larvae, 4 showed typical melanotic tumors while still in the second larval instar. This finding is of particular interest in view of the suggestion (BURNET and SANG 1964b; RIZKI 1960) that the second ecdysis has some special importance in tumor development; this is evidently not the case with the second instar tumors induced by FME. Cholesterol deficiency or supplementary tryptophan did not induce second instar tumors in this experiment, but their tumorigenic effects are not as marked as that of FME. The only other treatment which has induced second instar tumors in tu bw;+$^{su-tu}$ is the farnesoate derivative (LAW et al. 1966) which has this effect at concentrations of 0.07% wt/vol. and above (see Figure 9).

Time of tumor formation as influenced by genotype: Table 1 compares two tumor strains and the hybrid between them with respect to tumor expression and time of tumor formation when grown on standard medium. In this table, T1 and T50 are the times when the first tumor appears, and when 50% of the larvae have tumors, respectively, both corrected to a standard larval development time of 96 hrs. Tumor expression in tu55g is higher than in tu bw;+$^{su-tu}$, and the hybrid is intermediate between the two homozygotes in this respect. The table shows that genetically determined differences in tumor expression are associated with differences in time of tumor development, in the same way as the environmental effects mentioned above; that is, high tumor expression is associated with early onset of tumor appearance. However, animals of these genotypes do not form melanotic tumors before the third instar under control conditions.

TABLE 1

Tumor expression and time of tumor formation under standard conditions for three genotypes

Genotype	T1	T50	Final tumor expression
tu bw; +$^{su-tu}$	69	117	1.16
tu bw; +$^{su-tu}$ × tu 55g	69	88	2.40
tu55g	65	75	4.26

T1 = time of appearance of first tumor } all corrected to 96 hrs.
T50 = time when 50% of larvae have visible tumors } median pupation time.
(Based on sample sizes of 50–170)

139

TABLE 2

Effect of 4mM FME on tumor expression in various tumor strains

Strain	Tumor expression	
	Control	FME, 4mM
$tu\ bw;\ +^{su-tu}$	1.16	3.41*
$tu\ 55g$	2.71	6.98*
tu^K	0.196	2.99*
$tu^w\ rc$	1.04	2.25*

* Indicates tumors appeared in 2nd instar.

We have also investigated the effects of FME on some tumor genes other than *tu bw*. As Table 2 shows, FME at a level of 4mM can increase tumor expression in the *tu bw;+$^{su-tu}$*, *tu^K*, and *tu^{W}rc* strains, all of which carry non-allelic tumor genes, as well as in the *tu55g* strain, which has a tumor gene allelic with *tu bw* (ERK and SANG 1966). It is significant that, in all of these strains, FME induces tumors to form during the second instar. That is, the effect of FME in increasing tumor expression and inducing second instar tumors is not restricted to *tu bw* but extends to other allelic and non-allelic tumor genes.

By using the *tu55g* strain, which has a high control level of tumor expression, and which is particularly sensitive to FME treatment (Table 3), tumors have been induced to form during the first larval instar, in a few instances. This was accomplished by growing the larvae at 20°C, which can be regarded as a tumorigenic treatment (BRYANT 1967) on medium containing 6mM FME. The time course of tumor appearance in this population is shown in Figure 20; the maximum number of first instar larvae recorded as showing tumors was nine in a sample of 146, the T1 and T50 for tumor formation were 22 and 27 hrs, respectively (on a 96 hr development time scale), and the final tumor expression was 7.24. It has not proved possible to induce first instar tumors in the *tu bw;+$^{su-tu}$* strain, even by using 0.35% wt./vol. of the farnesoate derivative, which gave a tumor expression of 7.73. It seems, therefore, that tumor expression and time of tumor formation are somewhat independent in their genetic control. It is not possible with the data available to decide if the differences between the two strains,

TABLE 3

Effect of FME on tumor expression, and on the time of tumor formation, in the tu 55g *strain*

Treatment	Tumor expression	Tumors visible in second instar
Control	4.56	0
FME 0.5mM	4.56	0
FME 1mM	5.17	+
FME 2mM	6.08	+

in tumor expression and in time of tumor appearance, are due to differences in genetic background, or in the tumor locus itself.

Specificity of treatments which induce second instar tumors: It has been shown above that, under standard conditions, tumors are formed earlier in *tu55g* that in any of the other strains tested. This strain has therefore been used in experiments to determine if the induction of tumors during the second instar is a specific effect of juvenile hormone mimics, or alternatively, if the effect is shown by other potent tumorigenic treatments. Table 3 shows that tumors can be induced to form in the second instar by treatment with FME at a concentration of 1mM, but not at 0.5 mM. The value of tumor expression, above which tumors become visible in second instar larvae, is therefore between 4.56 and 5.17 for the *tu55g* strain. Attempts to exceed this level of expression have been made using a variety of tumorigenic treatments, and it is indeed possible to exceed it by the use of either of low temperature, or by replacing dietary cholesterol with dihydrocholesterol (shown to be tumorigenic by COOKE 1968). Low temperature gives a tumor expression of 5.87, and dihydrocholesterol gives 6.17, but in neither of these populations were tumors visible in second instar larvae. Therefore, second instar tumors are not merely a correlate of high tumor expression, but are a result of particular environmental treatments, namely potent juvenile hormone mimics such as FME and the farnesoate derivative.

Time of tumor formation in relation to developmental stage: All of the above observations of times of tumor formation were made on populations of larvae, and such experiments are limited in scope because the developmental stage of each larva is not known with precision. Hence these experiments cannot show if tumors appear at particular stages during each instar. This difficulty was overcome by growing larvae individually in separate tubes, and making observations at regular intervals of both instar changes and number of tumors present. The time of appearance of tumors was thus determined for each larva, in relation to the stage of development through each instar. Table 4 summarizes the results of such an experiment, using hybrid *tu bw;* $+^{su-tu} \times tu55g$ larvae grown on standard medium

TABLE 4

Time of tumor appearance in relation to developmental stage. Each larva grown individually on 0.1 ml defined medium. Strain tu bw; $+^{su-tu} \times$ tu55g

a) Average number of new tumors per individual which appear during developmental stages.

Diet	Number of larvae observed	First instar	Second instar			Third instar			Total	Tumor expression in adults
			Early	Mid	Late	Early	Mid	Late		
Control	74	0	0	0	0	0.12	0.16	1.68	1.96	2.40
4mM FME	57	0	1.10	0.91	0.67	0.56	0.47	0.60	4.31	4.18

b) Percentage of larvae at different developmental stages which have visible tumors.

Diet	Number of larvae observed	First instar	Second instar			Third instar			Penetrance in adults
			Early	Mid	Late	Early	Mid	Late	
Control	74	0	0	0	0	4.1	10.9	77.1	89.0
4mM FME	57	0	61.4	86.0	94.7	98.2	98.2	100.0	100.0

141

and on medium containing 4mM FME; this genotype, as noted before, gives a tumor expression and time of tumor formation which is intermediate between the two homozygotes. The time spent in each instar is divided into three parts, and the data are presented in two ways: first, the percentage of larvae showing tumors at each stage of development, and second, the average number of new tumors per larva which appear during each stage. On the standard medium, the majority of tumors do not become visible until the late third instar, as noted before, although some appear during the early and middle stages of the third instar. On FME-supplemented medium however, 61.4% of the larvae develop tumors early in the second instar, and tumors continue to appear in the treated group during the rest of the second and third instars. After the sudden onset of tumor appearance following the first ecdysis (which may be related to the liberation of haemocytes at this time) the rate of tumor formation during subsequent stages is fairly uniform, and tumors appear with only slightly decreasing probability during the early, middle and late second instar, and in early, middle and late third instar. That is, under these conditions the time of appearance of tumors is not closely related to the larval molting cycle, in contrast to the effects of the non-hormonal treatments studied by BURNET and SANG (1964b).

Table 4 also shows that the number of tumors appearing during the late third instar is greater in the control group than in the treated group. The early appearance of tumors in the treated group, therefore, seems to decrease the probability of late tumor appearance; this may be due to a decrease in the number of blood cells available for tumor formation, although observation of blood samples from highly tumorous larvae revealed no obvious deficiency of blood cells. The average number of tumors in the adults from the treated series in this experiment was slightly lower than the number developed by the larvae; GUÉLÉLOVITCH (1958) has also reported that the tumor frequency in adults of the *tu vg bw* strain is lower than that of pupae. These results indicate a resorption or, more likely, a fusion of tumors during the pupal phase. However in the control series, the number of tumors in adults is greater than that in larvae. This increase probably occurred in very late third instars (after the last observation before pupation), although we cannot exclude the possibility of tumor formation during metamorphosis.

DISCUSSION

The main conclusion from this study is that some substances which have juvenile hormone activity when tested in insects other than Diptera, are remarkably tumorigenic when fed to some melanotic tumor strains of Drosophila. Until there is an unequivocal demonstration that juvenile hormone acts in Diptera we cannot conclude that tumorigenesis is a direct consequence of juvenile hormone action, but it seems possible that this will prove to be so since the effects of the farnesoic acid derivative (BRYANT and SANG 1968; SPIELMAN and SKAFF 1967) and of natural juvenile hormone (SRIVASTAVA and GILBERT 1969) support the assumption that the hormonal control of development in Diptera is similar to that of other insects. And it would be surprising if this were not so.

142

The correlation found here is that compounds with high juvenile hormone activity in non-Dipteran insects increase the expression of the melanotic tumor gene in the *tu bw;+$^{su-tu}$* strain. Farnesyl methyl ether, dodecyl methyl ether and the derivative of farnesoic acid, all potent juvenile hormone mimics, are among the most active tumorigenic agents yet found. However, some related compounds which are less active, or inactive, as juvenile hormone mimics have no tumorigenic activity. For example, farnesene, tridecyl and tetradecyl methyl ether have no effect on tumorigenesis, while farnesol, nerolidol, farnesal, phytol, isophytol, pentadecyl methyl ether, geraniol and squalene actually reduce tumor frequency. There is one exception to the above generalisation; the butyl ethers of dodecanol and farnesol, which have negligible juvenile hormone activity (SCHNEIDERMAN *et al.* 1965), are as tumorigenic as the corresponding methyl ethers. This indicates that the specificity of the short chain of the molecule differs in its tumorigenic and its juvenile hormone functions, a conclusion which is reinforced by the finding that farnesyl diethylamine, whose juvenile hormone activity approaches that of farnesyl methyl ether, (SCHNEIDERMAN *et al.* 1965), actually reduces tumor expression. The specificity of the long chain of the molecule, on the other hand, is strikingly similar for the two activities, as is well demonstrated by the fact that dodecyl methyl ether has both tumorigenic and juvenile hormone activities, whereas tridecyl methyl ether has neither.

Although the correlation is not absolute, it seems reasonable to conclude that the tumorigenic effects reported here may be related to, or even due to, the high juvenile hormone activities of the materials concerned. The tumor-suppressing effects of the less active juvenile hormone mimics may be due to some other feature of the molecules, since some related materials with no juvenile hormone activity also show this effect.

These findings re-emphasize the conclusion, expressed by previous authors (BURDETTE 1954; BURNET and SANG 1964b; RIZKI 1960) that hormonal events are involved in melanotic tumor formation. But the nature of this involvement is far from clear. BURNET and SANG (1964b) discovered that the penetrance of the *tu bw* gene was modifiable by dietary treatments for only a short period which included the second larval molt, and furthermore that the haemocyte transformation leading to tumorigenesis was initiated in the time immediately following the dietary sensitive period. These authors, therefore, suggested that the tumor phenotype was due to an error in the reaction to hormonal changes at this time in development. The above evidence does not contradict this view, but it shows in addition that potent juvenile hormone mimics such as FME can cause tumor formation during earlier stages, which is unlikely to be related to humoral changes occurring at ecdyses. That is to say, tumorigenic treatments other than juvenile hormone mimics may indirectly affect the hormone balance at the second ecdysis, whereas FME for example may act directly on the haemocytes at any stage of development; larval molts would be of no special significance in the latter case. Unlike RIZKI (1960), we have been unable to find any abnormality of the ring gland of tumorous strains, which might explain why the second ecdysis is critical for the development of tumors in untreated larvae, or for the enhancement of

143

tumor frequency by dietary manipulations. The relative timing of larval and pupal molts is also normal in *tu bw* strains. Furthermore, we have been unable to induce melanotic tumor formation, using FME, in strains carrying no melanotic tumor genes. Therefore, it seems unlikely that melanotic tumors are merely the result of an endocrine abnormality which can be exaggerated or mimicked by feeding hormonally active materials. The genetic lesion in melanotic tumor strains must involve an abnormality of some system which is sensitive to the nutritional environment, and to the level of juvenile hormone. This implies, of course, that this system is normally regulated by the juvenile hormone, in which case it will be of obvious interest to examine the effects of the molting hormone, ecdysone, on melanotic tumor formation.

Thanks are due to the Agricultural Research Council and the Science Research Council for financial support, and to Miss MURIEL HASTINGS and Mrs. JUNE ATHERTON for technical assistance. Farnesol was obtained from the Aldrich Chemical Company, Inc.; nerolidol and phytol from K and K Laboratories, Ltd.; and dodecanol from the Sigma Chemical Company, Ltd. A sample of farnesoate derivative (LAW *et al.* 1966) was generously supplied by DR. FORBES W. ROBERTSON; pentadecyl methyl ether by DR. R. HOWE; isophytol, farnesal, farnesene, farnesyl and dodecyl butyl, and tridecyl and tetradecyl methyl ethers by DR. HOWARD A. SCHNEIDERMAN; and farnesyl methyl ether and farnesyl diethylamine by MESSRS. HOFFMAN LA ROCHE, Switzerland. The *tu bw*;$+^{su-tu}$ strain was kindly supplied by PROFESSOR BENTLEY GLASS.

LITERATURE CITED

BLOCH, K., 1965   The biological synthesis of cholesterol. Science **150**: 19–28.

Bowers, W. S., and M. J. Thompson, 1963 Juvenile hormone activity: effects of isoprenoid and straight-chain alcohols on insects. Science 142: 1469–1470.

Bryant, P. J., 1967 Ph.D. Thesis, University of Sussex.

Bryant, P. J., and J. H. Sang, 1968 Drosophila: lethal derangements of metamorphosis and modifications of gene expression caused by juvenile hormone mimics. Nature 220: 393–394.

Burdette, W. J., 1954 Effect of ligation of Drosophila larvae on tumor incidence. Cancer Res. 14: 780–782.

Burnet, B., and J. H. Sang, 1964a Physiological genetics of melanotic tumors in Drosophila melanogaster. II. The genetic basis of response to tumorigenic treatments in tu^K and $tu bw$; st su-tu strains. Genetics 49: 223–235. —— 1963b Physiological genetics of melanotic tumors in Drosophila melanogaster. III. Phenocritical period in relation to tumor formation in the tu bw; st su-tu strain. Genetics 49: 599–610.

Clayton, R. B., 1964 The utilisation of sterols by insects. J. Lipid Res. 5: 3–19.

Cooke, J., 1968 Ph.D. Thesis, University of Sussex.

Erk, F. C. and J. H. Sang, 1966 Allelism of second chromosome melanotic tumor genes. Drosophila Inform. Serv. 41: 95.

Glass, B., 1954 Drosophila Inform. Serv. 28: 74.

Glass, B., 1957 In pursuit of a gene. Science 126: 683–689.

Guélélovitch, S., 1958 Une tumeur héréditaire de la drosophile Drosophila melanogaster. Biologie méd. (Paris) 47: 711–810.

Jacobs, M. E., J. T. Bowman, and V. Walliser, 1958 Studies of a melanoma. Drosophila Inform. Serv. 32: 130.

Karlson, P., 1963 Chemistry and biochemistry of insect hormones. Angew. Chem., (International Edition in English) 2: 175–182.

Law, J. H., C. Yuan, and C. M. Williams, 1966 Synthesis of a material with high juvenile hormone activity. Proc. Natl. Acad. Sci. U.S. 55: 576–578.

Levinson, H. Z., 1966 Studies on the juvenile hormone (neotenin) activity of various hormonomimetic materials. Riv. Parassitol. 27: 47–63.

Oftedal, P., 1953 The histogenesis of a new tumor in Drosophila melanogaster, and a comparison with tumors of five other stocks. Z. Ind. Abst. Vererb. 85: 408–422.

Rizki, M. T. M., 1960 Melanotic tumor formation in Drosophila. J. Morphol. 106: 147–158.

Romaňuk, M., K. Sláma, and F. Šorm, 1967 Constitution of a compound with a pronounced juvenile hormone activity. Proc. Natl. Acad. Sci. U.S. 57: 349–352.

Sang, J. H., 1956 The quantitative nutritional requirements of Drosophila melanogaster. J. Exptl. Biol. 33: 45–72. —— 1966 Clearing Drosophila adults. Drosophila Inform. Serv. 41: 200.

Sang, J. H., and B. Burnet, 1963 Physiological genetics of melanotic tumors in Drosophila melanogaster. I. The effects of nutrient balance on tumor penetrance in the tu^K strain. Genetics 48: 235–253. —— 1967 Physiological genetics of melanotic tumors in Drosophila melanogaster. IV. Gene-environment interactions of tu-bw with different third chromosome backgrounds. Genetics 56: 743–754.

Schmialek, P., 1963 Über Verbindungen mit Juvenilhormonwirkung. Z. Naturforsch. 18b: 516–519.

Schneiderman, H. A., and L. I. Gilbert, 1964 Control of growth and development in insects. Science 143: 325–333.

SCHNEIDERMAN, H. A., A. KRISHNAKUMARAN, V. G. KULKARNI, and L. FRIEDMAN, 1965 Juvenile hormone activity of structurally unrelated compounds. J. Insect Physiol. 11: 1641–1649.

SPIELMAN, A., and V. SKAFF, 1967 Inhibition of metamorphosis and of ecdysis in mosquitoes. J. Insect Physiol. 13: 1087–1095.

SRIVASTAVA, U. S. and L. I. GILBERT, 1969 The influence of juvenile hormone on the metamorphosis of Sarcophaga bullata. J. Insect Physiol. 15: 177–189.

WIGGLESWORTH, V. B., 1963 The juvenile hormone effect of farnesol and some related compounds: quantitative experiments. J. Insect Physiol. 9: 105–119.

The Mechanism of Carcinogenesis
Investigated at the Molecular Level

Effects of 3-Methylcholanthrene Pretreatment on Microsomal Hydroxylation of 2-Acetamidofluorene by Various Rat Hepatomas

By PRABHAKAR D. LOTLIKAR

Many foreign compounds, including drugs and chemical carcinogens, are oxidized by liver microsomes of all animal species studied so far (Conney, 1967). Several transplantable rat tumours such as Morris hepatomas 5123C, 5123D and 7800 have been described as minimal deviation or well-differentiated hepatomas because they have many morphological and biochemical characteristics closely resembling normal liver; these hepatomas were initially produced by oral administration of various fluorene derivatives (Morris, 1965). These, as well as poorly differentiated and primary liver tumours, have low or negligible enzyme activity to oxidize foreign compounds (Conney, Brown, Miller & Miller, 1957; Neubert & Hoffmeister, 1960; Adamson & Fouts, 1961; Conney & Burns, 1963; Hart, Adamson, Morris & Fouts, 1965; Roger, Morris & Fouts, 1967). Conney & Burns (1963) have shown that hepatoma 5123C had low azo-dye N-demethylase enzyme activity and that this activity could be stimulated by administration of MC.* Phenobarbital pretreatment of tumour-bearing animals has also been shown to induce drug-

* Abbreviations: MC, 3-methylcholanthrene; AAF, 2-acetamidofluorene; x-hydroxy-AAF, 2-acetamido-x-hydroxyfluorene; 3′-methyl-DAB, 4-dimethylamino-3′-methylazobenzene.

metabolizing enzyme activities in several liver tumours (Hart et al. 1965; Roger et al. 1967).

N-Hydroxylation of AAF was first reported by Cramer, Miller & Miller (1960b). They showed that N-hydroxy-AAF appeared in the rat urine as a conjugate (probably the glucuronide) and was found in increasing amounts as the feeding of the carcinogen progressed. The potent carcinogen AAF is metabolized by rat liver microsomes, not only to various non-carcinogenic ring-hydroxylated products, namely 1-, 3-, 5- and 7-hydroxy-AAF (Booth & Boyland, 1957; Seal & Gutmann, 1959; Cramer, Miller & Miller, 1960a), but also to more carcinogenic N-hydroxy derivatives (Irving, 1964; Lotlikar, Enomoto, Miller & Miller, 1967). Administration of MC with AAF inhibits the carcinogenicity of AAF in the rat (Miyaji et al. 1953; Miller, Miller, Brown & MacDonald, 1958). Pretreatment of rats with MC also causes a decreased urinary excretion of N-hydroxy-AAF (Miller, Cramer & Miller, 1960; Lotlikar et al. 1967). However, in studies in vitro with rat liver microsomes, both ring and N-hydroxylation of AAF are increased severalfold when MC is administered to animals 24h before they are killed (Cramer et al. 1960a; Lotlikar et al. 1967). On the other hand, after pretreatment of hamsters with MC, there is a specific and relatively large increase only in N-hydroxylation by their liver microsomes (Lotlikar *et al.* 1967). From carbon monoxide inhibition studies it has been suggested that cytochrome P-450 is involved in ring hydroxylation and not in N-hydroxylation of aromatic amines (Kampffmeyer & Kiese, 1965; Hlavica & Kiese, 1969).

The purpose of the present work was to determine the N- and ring hydroxylation of AAF by microsomal preparations of various transplantable and primary hepatomas and their host livers with and without MC pretreatment of tumour-bearing animals.

MATERIALS AND METHODS

Animals. The slow growing well-differentiated Morris hepatomas 5123C, 5123D, 5123CTC and 7800 and poorly differentiated hepatomas 7288CTC were transplanted either intramuscularly or subcutaneously in Buffalo female rats. These tumour-bearing animals were kindly provided by Dr Harold P. Morris, School of Medicine, Howard University, Washington, D.C., U.S.A. The tumours were implanted in Washington and the tumour-bearing rats were shipped to Philadelphia, where they were maintained on a commercial diet until the tumours were large enough to use. The Novikoff hepatomas were propagated in Philadelphia by subcutaneous transplantation in female rats of Sprague–Dawley strain obtained from Holtzman Rat Co., Madison, Wis., U.S.A. The primary liver tumours were produced in adult male rats of CFN strain weighing 175–200g obtained from Carworth Farms Co., New City, N.Y., U.S.A., by feeding 0.06% 3′-methyl-DAB as described by Shatton, Donnelly & Weinhouse (1962). The primary mammary tumours were produced in adult Sprague–Dawley-strain female rats by oral administration of 10mg of MC/day for 20 consecutive days for a total of 200mg as described by Gruenstein, Meranze, Thatcher & Shimkin(1966). These mammary-tumour-bearing animals were kindly supplied by Mrs Margot Gruenstein of this Institute. Adult female Buffalo rats were used as control for these studies.

Chemicals. AAF was obtained from Mann Research Laboratories, New York, N.Y., U.S.A.; 3′-methyl-DAB and MC were purchased from Eastman Kodak Co., Rochester, N.Y., U.S.A. Authentic 1-, 3-, 5- and 7-hydroxy-AAF were kindly supplied by Dr James A. Miller, McArdle Laboratory for Cancer Research, University of Wisconsin, Madison, Wis., U.S.A. N-Hydroxy-AAF was prepared as described by Poirier, Miller & Miller (1963). NADH, NADPH and ATP were obtained from Sigma Chemical Co., St Louis, Mo., U.S.A. All other chemicals were of reagent grade.

Injection of MC. Animals were injected intraperitoneally with MC (10mg/100g body wt.) suspended in olive oil (10mg/ml) 24h before they were killed. Animals bearing primary tumours with 3′-methyl-DAB were fed on regular commercial diet for a week before MC injection. Control animals were injected with olive oil.

Preparation of microsomes. After the animals were decapitated, the tissues were immediately removed and chilled in ice-cold 0.25M-sucrose solution. Tumours were

then quickly freed from surrounding tissues and from necrotic material, if any. A 10% (w/v) homogenate of tissue prepared in 0.25M-sucrose solution was centrifuged at 8000g for 10min to remove nuclei and mitochondria. The microsomal pellet was obtained by centrifuging the mitochondrial supernatant at 105000g for 60min. The surface of the microsomal pellet was washed twice with 0.25M-sucrose before it was resuspended in the same medium.

Assay for ring and N-hydroxylation of AAF. The incubation medium contained 100μmol of potassium phosphate buffer, pH7.8, 400μmol of KCl, 240μmol of nicotinamide, 600μmol of KF, 4μmol of ATP, 1.06μmol of NADPH, 1.22μmol of NADH, 0.45μmol of AAF added in 0.2ml of methanol, tissue microsomes equivalent to 60mg wet wt. of tissue, 150μmol of sucrose and water to a final volume of 6.0ml. This incubation medium is almost identical with that described by Cramer *et al.* (1960a) for ring hydroxylation of AAF except for the addition of KF. The presence of 0.1M-KF in the incubation system inhibits deacetylase activity (Seal & Gutmann, 1959; Irving, 1964; Lotlikar, Miller, Miller & Margreth, 1965). The flasks were incubated in air for 20min at 37°C, after which 8ml of ice-cold-1M-sodium acetate buffer, pH6.0, was added per flask. Contents of 18 flasks were combined for each analysis and extracted immediately with diethyl ether. The acidic metabolites were extracted from the ether extract into 0.5M-NaOH; finally the alkali extract was neutralized to pH6.0 and the metabolites were extracted in diethyl ether. The acidic metabolites were chromatographed on Whatman no. 1 paper with cyclohexane-2-methylpropan-2-ol-acetic acid-water(16:4:2:1, by vol.) (Weisburger, Weisburger, Morris & Sober, 1956). After chromatography the strips were air-dried and then viewed under u.v. light. Appropriate absorption zones were cut out and eluted overnight in 3ml of 95% (v/v) ethanol. The metabolites were determined quantitatively by u.v. absorption in the range 350–270nm by using a Hitachi–Coleman recording spectrophotometer. The following molar extinction coefficients with maximum wavelengths in parentheses were used for authentic hydroxy compounds of AAF: N-hydroxy-AAF, 23400 (287nm); 3-hydroxy-AAF, 17400 (315nm); 5-hydroxy-AAF, 25500 (283nm); 7-hydroxy-AAF, 29800 (291nm). Before spectral analysis, the N-hydroxy-AAF was separated from AAF by extraction with 0.5M-NaOH. All of the results presented were corrected by the following recovery data: N-hydroxy-AAF, 75%; 3-hydroxy-AAF, 70%; 5-hydroxy-AAF, 90%; 7-hydroxy-AAF, 63%. The amounts of 1-hydroxy-AAF were generally too low to measure adequately and the values for this metabolite have therefore been omitted. Wherever values of 10 or less nmol/20min per g wet wt. of tissue are given for any metabolite, it indicates that a small amount of u.v.-light-absorbing material with a non-characteristic spectrum was eluted.

RESULTS

Rates of both N- and ring hydroxylation of AAF by liver and kidney microsomes from normal rats with and without MC pretreatment are presented in Table 1. The liver of untreated control animals has much greater hydroxylating activity than has

149

Table 1. *Effects of MC pretreatment on the N- and ring hydroxylation of AAF by liver and kidney microsomes from control rats*

Adult female Buffalo strain rats weighing 200–250 g were used in these experiments. Other details are as described in the Materials and Methods section. Results are given as means ±s.e.m. of determinations of four animals.

			Hydroxylation (nmol formed/20 min per g wet wt. of tissue)			
Tissue		MC pretreatment	N-Hydroxy-AAF	3-Hydroxy-AAF	5-Hydroxy-AAF	7-Hydroxy-AAF
Liver		−	25± 8	13± 2	17± 3	115± 10
		+	139±31	204±70	251±75	748±184
Kidney		−	9± 3	5± 2	2± 1	4± 1
		+	10± 2	28± 8	19± 3	65± 14

Table 2. *Effects of MC pretreatment on N- and ring hydroxylation of AAF by well-differentiated rat hepatomas and the host liver and kidney*

All details are described in the Materials and Methods section. Results are given as means±s.e.m.

				Hydroxylation (nmol formed/20 min per g wet wt. of tissue)			
Tissue	Rat tumour	MC pretreatment	No. of analyses	N-hydroxy-AAF	3-Hydroxy-AAF	5-Hydroxy-AAF	7-Hydroxy-AAF
Liver	5123D	−	4	16± 6	7± 5	11± 3	23± 11
		+	2	46± 3	139±28	282± 4	453± 39
Tumour		−	4	4± 3	3± 1	6± 2	10± 4
		+	2	9± 1	90± 7	93±16	152± 14
Liver	5123C	−	4	18± 2	6± 3	10± 2	18± 5
		+	2	156±46	152±42	335±55	512±112
Kidney		−	4	6± 2	10± 3	8± 1	10± 5
		+	2	3± 1	48± 5	23± 6	49± 11
Tumour		−	5	10± 6	2± 2	5± 5	6± 4
		+	2	13± 3	85± 5	70±10	129± 9
Liver	5123CTC	−	2	11± 3	6± 1	15± 4	21± 5
		+	2	43±17	133± 4	141± 3	228± 42
Tumour		−	2	9± 4	11± 4	15± 5	11± 2
		+	2	37± 7	82± 4	59± 3	93± 10
Liver	7800	−	2	16± 3	3± 2	13± 2	25± 13
		+	4	88±16	184±48	152±10	290± 69
Tumour		−	2	7± 3	6± 1	7± 3	10± 1
		+	4	6± 2	36±10	28± 7	52± 7

kidney. Pretreatment of animals with MC increased both N- and ring hydroxylating activity of liver several-fold. Similar results were obtained with weanling male rats (Lotlikar *et al.* 1967). Activity in the kidney of treated animals showed several-fold increase in ring hydroxylation without affecting concentrations of N-hydroxy-AAF. The enzyme activities in kidney after MC stimulation were much less than in liver. Wattenberg & Leong (1962) and Gelboin & Blackburn (1964) have also reported increases in benzpyrene hydroxylase in kidney extracts after MC pretreatment of animals.

The activities of various well-differentiated hepatomas and their host livers are summarized in Table 2. Tumour tissues and livers of all untreated tumour-bearing rats had low hydroxylating activity;

activity of the livers was higher than that of tumours. Pretreatment with MC caused several-fold increase in both N- and ring hydroxylation in the host livers, whereas in tumours except 5123CTC it caused a many-fold increase in ring hydroxylation only. Tumour 5123CTC showed a fourfold increase in N-hydroxylation activity also. Kidneys of the tumour-bearing rats also responded to MC pretreatment, like kidneys of non-tumour-bearing rats (see Table 1).

The effects of MC administration on the rates of AAF hydroxylation by poorly differentiated rat hepatomas and their host livers are given in Table 3. Host livers of untreated rats bearing 7288CTC tumour formed much greater amounts of N- and ring-hydroxylated products of AAF compared with

Table 3. *Hydroxylation of AAF by poorly differentiated rat hepatomas and the host liver with and without MC pretreatment*

All details are as described in the Materials and Methods Section. Values are given as means±s.e.m. of three determinations.

			Hydroxylation (nmol formed/20 min per g wet wt. of tissue)			
Tissue	Rat tumour	MC pretreatment	N-Hydroxy-AAF	3-Hydroxy-AAF	5-Hydroxy-AAF	7-Hydroxy-AAF
Liver	7288CTC	−	89 ± 29	120 ± 20	113 ± 10	249 ± 33
		+	83 ± 17	146 ± 6	202 ± 13	609 ± 17
Tumour		−	11 ± 3	4 ± 1	7 ± 2	5 ± 3
		+	9 ± 2	5 ± 2	6 ± 3	8 ± 5
Liver	Novikoff	−	8 ± 3	5 ± 2	12 ± 4	52 ± 12
		+	14 ± 5	102 ± 12	314 ± 62	456 ± 87
Tumour		−	6 ± 2	2 ± 1	5 ± 2	6 ± 1
		+	8 ± 3	5 ± 1	6 ± 3	6 ± 2

Table 4. *Effects of MC pretreatment on hydroxylation of AAF by primary tumours and the host tissues*

The primary liver tumours were produced in adult male rats weighing 175–200 g by administration of 0.06% 3'-methyl-DAB for 17 weeks as described by Shatton et al. (1962). These animals were fed on regular commerical diet for a week before MC injection. The primary mammary tumours were produced in adult Sprague–Dawley-strain female rats by oral administration of 10 mg of MC/day for 20 days. All other details are described in the Materials and Methods Section. Values are given as means±s.e.m. of three determinations.

			Hydroxylation (nmol formed/20 min per g wet wt. of tissue)			
Tissue	Rat tumour	MC pretreatment	N-Hydroxy-AAF	3-Hydroxy-AAF	5-Hydroxy-AAF	7-Hydroxy-AAF
Liver	Liver	−	19 ± 1	13 ± 3	8 ± 4	30 ± 15
		+	16 ± 3	112 ± 62	104 ± 14	373 ± 147
Tumour		−	8 ± 3	6 ± 2	3 ± 2	7 ± 3
		+	6 ± 2	25 ± 2	11 ± 5	44 ± 3
Liver	Mammary	−	10 ± 2	27 ± 6	10 ± 3	31 ± 13
		+	28 ± 4	127 ± 3	123 ± 19	218 ± 24
Tumour		−	9 ± 1	2 ± 1	8 ± 3	3 ± 1
		+	6 ± 2	3 ± 2	16 ± 3	7 ± 4
Kidney		−	10 ± 4	5 ± 2	8 ± 1	6 ± 2
		+	7 ± 2	42 ± 9	38 ± 7	50 ± 18

host livers of Novikoff or well-differentiated-tumour bearing rats (see Table 1). Pretreatment of 7288CTC-tumour-bearing rats with MC increased the formation of 7- and 5-hydroxy-AAF by the liver about twofold without affecting the amounts of N- and 3-hydroxy-AAF. On the other hand, MC pretreatment of rats bearing Novikoff tumour caused several-fold increase in ring hydroxylation, i.e. formation of 7-, 5- and 3-hydroxy-AAF, by their livers without appreciably affecting amounts of N-hydroxy-AAF. Hydroxylating activities of both types of tumours were low and they could not be altered by MC pretreatment of animals.

The results presented above were obtained only with transplanted hepatomas. It was important to investigate whether hydroxylating activities of primary tumours could be altered by MC pretreatment of tumour-bearing animals. Results obtained with primary hepatomas produced by

3'-methyl-DAB and mammary tumours produced by MC are presented in Table 4. Hydroxylation of AAF by liver from both groups of tumour-bearing animals could be increased several-fold by MC administration. Hepatoma showed an increase in ring-hydroxylating activity on MC pretreatment, whereas mammary tumour was unresponsive.

DISCUSSION

The above results show a great variation in AAF-hydroxylating activities of various tumours and their host livers on MC pretreatment of animals. Host livers of all tumour bearing animals except those with tumour 7288CTC demonstrated low hydroxylating ability, which could be stimulated several-fold by administration of MC 24h before the animals were killed.

Prior or simultaneous administration of ethionine,

puromycin or actinomycin D with either MC or phenobarbital prevents the stimulation of microsomal oxidative enzymes (Conney, Miller & Miller, 1957; Conney, Davison, Gastel & Burns, 1960; Gelboin & Blackburn, 1964; Lotlikar et al. 1967). These and amino acid-incorporation studies (Gelboin & Blackburn, 1963) indicate that MC, phenobarbital and several other inducers (Conney, 1967) cause induction or synthesis of new microsomal enzyme proteins.

It has been shown that several well-differentiated tumours, namely Morris hepatomas 5123C, 5123D and 7800, have either little or no ability to metabolize various drugs (Conney & Burns, 1963; Hart et al. 1965; Lotlikar et al. 1965; Roger et al. 1967). The present results are in agreement with these earlier findings. Pretreatment of animals with MC caused several-fold increase in the hydroxylating activities of tumours compared with the tumours of untreated animals. These stimulations are much more pronounced than those observed with phenobarbital treatment (Hart et al. 1965; Roger et al. 1967). In the present experiments only one tumour, Morris hepatoma 5123CTC, could N-hydroxylate AAF when tumour-bearing animals were pretreated with MC. This appears to be the first example of N-hydroxylation of AAF by any tumour tissue studied so far. The present results suggest that the activities of oxidative enzymes are low or diminished in well-differentiated tumours, but that the enzyme activities can be increased in these tumours by certain inducers such as MC.

In contrast with well-differentiated hepatomas, poorly differentiated hepatomas could not be stimulated by MC pretreatment. Thus, in my experiments, both tumours 7288CTC and Novikoff were resistant to MC effect. Hart et al. (1965) observed that pretreatment of Novikoff-tumour-bearing animals with phenobarbital did not have any effect on the metabolism of aminopyrine, neoprontosil or p-nitrobenzoic acid by a supernatant fraction from the Novikoff hepatoma. They reported, however, that the side-chain oxidation of hexobarbital was stimulated in this tumour to a slight but statistically significant extent. It appears that various substrates have different affinities for the oxidative enzymes. In the present studies, host liver of 7288CTC-tumour-bearing animals had high N- and ring-hydroxylating activity before MC pretreatment. Administration of MC increased the activity about twofold. One possible explanation for the high activity in the host liver before MC pretreatment could be that the tumour might have acted as an inducer for the host liver.

Conney & Burns (1963) reported that MC pretreatment was unable to induce the synthesis of the azo-dye N-demethylase system in a primary hepatoma produced by 3'-methyl-DAB administration. Hart et al. (1965) also demonstrated that phenobarbital pretreatment of animals did not appear to stimulate aminopyrine demethylation by primary liver tumours produced by DAB administration. However, they observed that the metabolism of hexobarbital by these primary tumours was stimulated to some extent. In the present studies, primary hepatoma produced by 3'-methyl-DAB was stimulated to some degree on MC pretreatment. No stimulation could be observed with primary mammary tumour produced by MC administration.

After pretreatment of animals with MC, the relatively specific and large increase in N-hydroxylation by hamster liver microsomes, compared with the relatively small increase in N-hydroxylation and large increase in ring hydroxylation by rat liver microsomes under similar conditions, suggested that MC treatment might affect carcinogenesis by AAF differently in the two species (Lotlikar et al. 1967). The work of Enomoto, Miyake & Sato (1968) supports this hypothesis. They demonstrated that, compared with the marked inhibition of AAF carcinogenesis in rats by MC administration (Miller et al. 1958; Miyaji et al. 1953), no inhibition of tumour induction by AAF was obtained on simultaneous administration of MC to hamsters. In the present experiments, tumours when stimulated followed the hydroxylation pattern of rat liver and not of hamster liver. These studies suggest that some of the control mechanisms (induction with MC) that are present in normal liver are still functional in well-differentiated tumours but are apparently lost in poorly differentiated hepatomas.

The present studies demonstrated that, in addition to liver, kidneys of tumour-bearing animals could be easily stimulated by MC pretreatment. Wattenberg & Leong (1962) and Gelboin & Blackburn (1964) have also reported such stimulatory effects of MC on benzpyrene hydroxylase in rat liver, kidney, small intestine, lungs and several other tissues.

This investigation was supported by a Career Development Award (5-KO4-CA42362) and a research grant (CA-10604) from the National Cancer Institute, U.S. Public Health Service. The excellent technical assistance of Mrs Manjula Chandu Lal is greatefully acknowledged.

REFERENCES

Adamson, R. H. & Fouts, J. R. (1961). Cancer Res. 21, 667.
Booth, J. & Boyland, E. (1957). Biochem. J. 66, 73.
Conney, A. H. (1967). Pharmac. Rev. 19, 317.
Conney, A. H., Brown, R. R., Miller, J. A. & Miller, E. C. (1957). Cancer Res. 17, 628.
Conney, A. H. & Burns, J. J. (1963). In Advances in Enzyme Regulation, vol. 1, p. 189. Edited by Weber, G. Oxford: Pergamon Press Ltd.

Conney, A. H., Davison, C., Gastel, R. & Burns, J. J. (1960). *J. Pharmac. exp. Ther.* **130**, 1.

Conney, A. H., Miller, E. C. & Miller, J. A. (1957). *J. biol. Chem.* **228**, 753.

Cramer, J. W., Miller, J. A. & Miller, E. C. (1960a). *J. biol. Chem.* **235**, 250.

Cramer, J. W., Miller, J. A. & Miller, E. C. (1960b). *J. biol. Chem.* **235**, 885.

Enomoto, M., Miyake, M. & Sato, K. (1968). *Gann.* **59**, 177.

Gelboin, H. V. & Blackburn, N. R. (1963). *Biochim. biophys. Acta*, **72**, 657.

Gelboin, H. V. & Blackburn, N. R. (1964). *Cancer Res.* **24**, 356.

Gruenstein, M., Meranze, D., Thatcher, D. & Shimkin, M. B. (1966). *J. natn. Cancer Inst.* **36**, 483.

Hart, L. G., Adamson, R. H., Morris, H. P. & Fouts, J. R. (1965). *J. Pharmac. exp. Ther.* **149**, 7.

Hlavica, P. & Kiese, M. (1969). *Biochem. Pharmac.* **18**, 1501.

Irving, C. C. (1964). *J. biol. Chem.* **239**, 1589.

Kampffmeyer, P. & Kiese, M. (1965). *Arch. exp. Path. Pharmak.* **250**, 1.

Lotlikar, P. D., Enomoto, M., Miller, J. A. & Miller, E. C. (1967). *Proc. Soc. exp. Biol. Med.* **125**, 341.

Lotlikar, P. D., Miller, E. C. Miller, J. A. & Margreth, A. (1965). *Cancer Res.* **25**, 1743.

Miller, E. C., Miller, J. A., Brown, R. R. & MacDonald, J. C. (1958). *Cancer Res.* **18**, 469.

Miller, J. A., Cramer, J. W. & Miller, E. C. (1960). *Cancer Res.* **20**, 950.

Miyaji, T., Moskowski, L. I., Senoo, T., Ogata, M., Odo, T., Kawai, K., Sayama, Y., Ishida, H. & Matsuo, H. (1953). *Gann.* **44**, 281.

Morris, H. P. (1965). *Adv. Cancer Res.* **9**, 227.

Neubert, D. & Hoffmeister, I. (1960). *Arch. exp. Path. Pharmak.* **239**, 234.

Poirier, L. A., Miller, J. A. & Miller, E. C. (1963). *Cancer Res.* **23**, 790.

Roger, L. A., Morris, H. P. & Fouts, J. R. (1967). *J. Pharmac. exp. Ther.* **157**, 227.

Seal, U. S. & Gutmann, H. R. (1959). *J. biol. Chem.* **234**, 648.

Shatton, J. B., Donnelly, A. J. & Weinhouse, S. (1962). *Cancer Res.* **22**, 1372.

Wattenburg, L. W. & Leong, J. L. (1962). *J. Histochem. Cytochem.* **10**, 412.

Weisburger, J. H., Weisburger, E. K., Morris, H. P. & Sober, H. A. (1956). *J. natn. Cancer Inst.* **17**, 363.

153

Respiration and Glycolysis of Cells Transformed with 4-Nitroquinoline-1-Oxide and Its Derivative (34776)

KIYOMI SATO, TOSHIO KUROKI, AND HARUO SATO
(Introduced by I. Yamane)

An increased aerobic glycolysis (1, 2, 4) and an inhibition of respiration by glucose addition [the Crabtree effect] (3) are the most commonly reported alterations in malignant cells. This increased aerobic glycolysis is observed not only in many established strains induced by chemical carcinogens *in vivo* but also in transformed cells induced by viruses *in vitro* (5–8) as well as *in vivo* (9–10).

Recently in our laboratory, a transformation system for hamster embryonic cells (HE cells) with 4-nitroquinoline-1-oxide and its derivatives was established (11, 12). Therefore, an attempt to compare the glucose metabolism of nontreated HE cells with that of these transformants was made to observe if an increase in aerobic glycolysis and appearance of the Crabtree effect would be accompanied with even *in vitro* chemical carcinogenesis.

Materials and Methods. Three transformants from HE cells and nontreated HE cells, as control cells, were used in this study. Histories and characteristics of the cells are summarized in Table I. The detailed methods and procedures of transformation were described elsewhere (12). The culture medium consisted of Eagle's minimum essential medium supplemented with 1 mM pyruvate, 0.2 mM serine, and 10% calf serum. The exponentially growing cells (5–10 $\times$ 10^7 cells cultured in 6–8 Roux bottles) were harvested with 0.025% pronase in PBS, followed by washing twice with Krebs-Ringer-phosphate buffer (pH 7.4) (Ca^{2+}-free), packed by centrifugation at 600g for 2 min, and resuspended in the same buffer. Incubation was carried out in air according to the procedures described elsewhere (13). Oxygen consumption was measured manometrically. The production of $^{14}CO_2$ was measured as described by Tsuiki and Kikuchi (14). Lactate was determined by the method of Barker and Summerson (15).

Results and Discussion. The results of representative experiments are presented in Table II. When no substrate was added, oxygen consumption (endogenous respiration) was lower in the transformants than in the control cells. In the transformants, the rate of the endogenous respiration declined with time, apparently owing to decrease of endogenous substrates. In the presence of pyruvate, a fuel substance of the TCA cycle, oxygen consumption continued to proceed at a constant rate, and was higher in transformants than in control cells, suggesting that respiratory capacity was not reduced in these transformants. In virus-transformed cells, the reduction of respiration was described in some reports (5, 10), but was not observed in another report (6). Accordingly, this phenomenon seems to be not so characteristic of malignant cells as compared with an increase in aerobic glycolysis described below. When exogenous substrates were absent, the transformants except for NQ-19/Clone 4 did not

TABLE I. Summary of the Histories and Characteristics of the Cells Used.

Cells	Carcinogens[a]	Days and generations after treatment with carcinogen	Malignancy (stage)[b]
HE	None	12 days, 3 gen.	—
HA-7	$10^{-5}M$ 4HAQO	142 days, 7 gen.	+ (M2)
HA-2	$10^{-5}M$ 4HAQO	118 days, 12 gen.	+ (M3)
NQ-19/Cl.4	$10^{-6}M$ 4NQO	163 days, 17 gen.	+ (M3)

[a] 4HAQO: 4-hydroxyaminoquinoline-1-oxide HCl; 4NQO: 4-nitroquinoline-1-oxide.
[b] M1, M2, and M3 indicate the stage of malignancy of transformed cells. At stage M2, the tumor developed progressively after a long latent period after host transplantation, while at stage M3, the tumor growth began soon after the transplantation and never regressed. Details were reported elsewhere (12).

156

TABLE II. Oxygen Consumption and Glucose Metabolism of HE Cells and the Transformants.[a]

		HE cells	HA-7	HA-2	NQ-19/Cl.4
O₂ consumed	None (1)	2.37	1.85	1.61	1.33
	Glucose (2)	2.35	1.92	2.03	1.18
	Pyruvate (3)	2.53	2.34	3.00	NE[b]
	Glucose, pyruvate (4)	2.62	2.18	2.24	NE
Crabtree effect	(2)/(1)	1.00	1.04	1.25	0.89
	(4)/(3)	1.03	0.93	0.74	/
Lactate formed	Glucose	1.30	3.16	8.77	8.35
¹⁴CO₂ formed	Glucose-1-¹⁴C	0.069	0.064	0.125	0.091
	Glucose-6-¹⁴C	0.015	0.015	0.040	0.020
	6-C/1-C	0.22	0.23	0.32	0.22

[a] All the substrates were 10 mM; the values are expressed as μmoles/hr/10 mg dry weight (about 2 × 10⁷ cells).
[b] Not estimated.

157

exhibit the Crabtree effect. This is probably due to the low endogenous respiration in these cells, since the typical Crabtree effect was observed in the presence of pyruvate. The control cells did not show this effect in the presence as well as absence of pyruvate. Of the data shown in Table II, the most remarkable change observed in the transformants was an increase in aerobic glycolysis: aerobic lactate production was 3–9 μmoles for the transformants as compared with 1.3 μmoles for the control cells under the same conditions. In addition, the rate seemed to be correlated with the grade of malignancy. The $^{14}CO_2$ ratio of C-6:C-1 has been considered as a useful index for the evaluation of the participation of the TCA cycle or the pentose phosphate shunt in total glucose oxidation. The ratio is known to decrease in many tumors [suggesting greater participation of the shunt] (16). In our experiments, the ratio found for HE cells was low, and no significant difference was observed between the control cells and the transformants. Under comparable conditions, Ehrlich ascites tumor (13) and Yoshida ascites hepatomas (17) gave values ranging from 0.05 to 0.01. The ratio found for the *in vitro* transformants are, thus, higher than those for the ascites hepatomas, and this could be related to the lower inhibition of respiration by glucose in these transformants as compared with the ascites tumors.

Although the increased aerobic glycolysis is reported to be a characteristic of many malignant cell strains, its significance has been in much dispute. However, there are some reports which suggest that the rate of glycolysis increases with the rate of cell multiplication in virus-transformed cells (7, 8) as well as in transplantable rat hepatomas (18–20). Our experiments show that the transformation and development of malignancy induced *in vitro* with the chemical carcinogens are accompanied by an increase in aerobic glycolysis. Furthermore, the increase

158

appears to be correlated with the grade of malignancy. Thus, the results may support the view (5–8) that the increased aerobic glycolysis can be a simple biochemical indicator of neoplastic conversion.

In the present experiments, the need for relatively large amounts of the transformed cells made it unable to use them in the earliest stage. If aerobic glycolysis increases as a sole consequence of long-term culture, there still remains the possibility that the transformation by the chemical carcinogens is not a sole cause of increased aerobic glycolysis reported above. However, Sanford et al. (7) reported that the glycolytic activities of the untreated hamster embryo cells did not increase at least until the 240th culture day. As the cells used in our experiments were maintained under similar conditions, the increased aerobic glycolysis could be attributed to the treatment with chemical carcinogens.

Summary. Hamster embryonic cells transformed *in vitro* with 4-nitroquinoline-1-oxide and its derivative exhibited an increased aerobic glycolysis and an inhibition of respiration by glucose addition in the presence of pyruvate (the Crabtree effect). These changes, which are known to be characteristic of many malignant cells strains, appear to be correlated with the grade of malignancy.

1. Warburg, O., Biochem. Z. 142, 317 (1923).
2. Aisenberg, A. C., "The Glycolysis and Respiration of Tumors," p. 1. Academic Press, New York (1961).

3. Aisenberg, A. C., "The Glycolysis and Respiration of Tumors," p. 172. Academic Press, New York (1961).

4. Wenner, C. E., Advan. Enzymol. **29**, 322 (1967).

5. Morgan, H. R., and Gonapathy, S., Proc. Soc. Exp. Biol. Med. **113**, 312 (1963).

6. Paul, J., Broadfood, M. M., and Walker, P., Int. J. Cancer **1**, 207 (1966).

7. Sanford, K. K., Barker, B. E., Woods, M. W., Parshad, R., and Law, L. W., J. Nat. Cancer Inst. **39**, 705 (1967).

8. Temin, H. M., Int. J. Cancer **3**, 273 (1968).

9. Burk, D., Sprince, H., Spangler, J. M., Kabat, E. A., Furth, J., and Claude, A., J. Nat. Cancer Inst. **2**, 201 (1941).

10. Levine, A. S., Stricker, F., Uhl, R., and Ashmore, J., Nature (London) **188**, 229 (1960).

11. Sato, H., and Kuroki, T., Proc. Jap. Acad. **42**, 1211 (1966).

12. Kuroki, T., and Sato, H., J. Nat. Cancer Inst. **41**, 53 (1968).

13. Sato, K., Suzuki, R., and Tsuiki, S., Biochim. Biophys. Acta **165**, 189 (1968).

14. Tsuiki, S., and Kikuchi, G., Biochim. Biophys. Acta **64**, 514 (1962).

15. Barker, S. B., and Summerson, W. H., J. Biol. Chem. **138**, 535 (1941).

16. Aisenberg, A. C., "The Glycolysis and Respiration of Tumors," p. 92. Academic Press, New York (1961).

17. Takeda, H., and Tsuiki, S., GANN **58**, 221 (1967).

18. Burk, D., Woods, M., and Hunter, J., J. Nat. Cancer Inst. **38**, 839 (1967).

19. Weber, G., GANN Monogr. **1**, 151 (1966).

20. Weinhouse, S., GANN Monogr. **1**, 99 (1966).

STUDIES ON CARCINOGEN-BINDING PROTEINS

I. ISOLATION AND CHARACTERIZATION OF AMINOAZO DYE-BOUND PROTEIN AFTER ADMINISTRATION OF A SINGLE LARGE DOSE OF 3'-METHYL-4-DIMETHYLAMINOAZOBENZENE TO RATS

TSUTOMU SUGIMOTO AND HIROSHI TERAYAMA

INTRODUCTION

Carcinogenic aminoazo dye can bind to cellular proteins[1] in the target tissue as can other chemical carcinogens[2-5]. Using the 105 000 × g supernatant fraction from the liver of rats which had been fed a diet containing 3'-methyl-4-dimethylamino-

Abbreviations: 3'-MDAB, 3'-methyl-4-dimethylaminoazobenzene; 2-MDAB, 2-methyl-4-dimethylaminoazobenzene.

161

azobenzene (3'-MDAB) for 18–20 days, Soʀᴏғ et al.[6] reported that most of the dye-binding protein was recovered in a specific narrow band that was separated by zone electrophoresis in veronal buffer (pH 8.6). The slowly migrating band thus separated was named "slow h_2" and seemed to consist of proteins of somewhat basic nature. By means of gel filtration on Sephadex G-200, Soʀᴏғ et al.[7-9] found that the dye-binding protein in the slow-h_2 fraction had the molecular weight of 60 000–80 000. In addition to this dye-binding protein, they also indicated the presence of minor dye-binding proteins having molecular weights of 30 000–40 000 and 10 000–15 000, respectively. On the other hand, Kᴇᴛᴛᴇʀᴇʀ et al.[10] recently investigated the isolation of dye-binding protein from the liver of rats given a single large dose of 3'-MDAB and succeeded in isolating a basic dye-binding protein having the molecular weight of 45 000 and the isoelectric point of 8.4. They also reported the presence of two low-molecular-weight proteins (14 000) having isoelectric points near neutrality.

No systematic study has been carried out to elucidate the cause of the discrepancy concerning the nature of dye-binding proteins between the two research techniques: continuous feeding[7-9] and a single large dose administration[10].

In this paper the authors report on the isolation of aminoazo dye-binding proteins from the liver of rats given carcinogenic 3'-MDAB and noncarcinogenic (or very slightly carcinogenic[11]) 2-MDAB each in a single large dose with special attention to the possible identity of the dye-binding proteins with liver arginase, as suggested by Soʀᴏғ et al.[8]. Contrary to the results of previous investigators, we found that the carcinogenic aminoazo dye is bound preferentially to nonbasic protein (Fraction I) and to a less extent to slightly basic protein (Fraction IV). The binding to slightly more basic proteins (Fractions VI and VII), which seem to correspond to the slow h_2 proteins in the cell sap of the rat liver, was relatively less after the administration of a single large dose. In contrast with 3'-MDAB, the binding of 2-methyl-4-dimethyl-aminoazobenzene (2-MDAB) to the Fraction I proteins (nonbasic) was rather small and the dye was preferentially bound to the Fraction IV proteins.

METHODS AND MATERIALS

Male Wistar rats were given 40 mg of 3'-MDAB or 2-MDAB dissolved in olive oil through a stomach tube. The rats were killed after 40 h and the livei was perfused *in situ* with cold 0.25 M sucrose. The 50% liver homogenate prepared in 0.25 M sucrose was centrifuged at 10 000 × g for 20 min, and the supernatant was centrifuged again at 105 000 × g for 2 h. The final supernatant is referred to as the rat liver cell sap, and was used as the starting material for the purification of dye-binding proteins.

Chromatography on CM-cellulose was carried out by using a column of 2 cm × 26 cm which had been equilibrated with 0.01 M Tris–HCl buffer (pH 7.0). Elution was carried out by running 0.01 M Tris–HCl buffer (pH 7.0), 0.01, 0.02 and 0.05 M NaCl in the same buffer, successively. Gel filtration on Sephadex G-100 (or G-200) was carried out by using a column of 2.8 cm × 62 cm and 0.1 M KCl in 0.05 M Tris–HCl buffer (pH 7.5) as solvent at the flow rate of 20 ml/h. In both chromatographies fractions of 5.5 ml effluent were collected. Molecular weights of dye-binding proteins were estimated from elution volumes of the dye-binding proteins in Sephadex G-100 or G-200 gel filtration. Standard proteins of known molecular weights, such as bovine liver arginase, bovine serum albumin or cytochrome c, were subjected to the gel filtration for this purpose.

Electrophoresis of the dye-binding proteins was carried out on strips of cellulose acetate (cellogel) in 0.07 M veronal buffer (pH 8.6) or in 0.01 M Tris–HCl buffer of pH 6.05 and 4.90, respectively, for 90 min under the conditions of 0.75 mA/cm and 12 V/cm. After the run the strips were dipped into 1% amido black 10B or 10% trichloroacetic acid in 50% ethanol to stain protein or protein-bound dye, respectively.

Protein was assayed according to LOWRY et al.[12]. The protein-bound dye was estimated spectrophotometrically in concentrated formic acid. The protein was first precipitated with trichloroacetic acid, washed thoroughly with a chloroform–methanol (3:1, v/v) mixture and then dissolved in formic acid. The molar extinction coefficient of $4 \cdot 10^4$ was assumed for the maximal Q-band absorption of protein-bound dye. Arginase activity was assayed by the method of VAN SLYKE AND ARCHIBALD[13]. One unit of arginase was defined as the enzyme activity that generated 1 μmole urea per min under the assay conditions.

. Preparation of the polar dye from dye-bound proteins was carried out by the method of TERAYAMA[14] using a large excess of pronase. The polar dye in 2 M HCl was washed with ethyl acetate, and chromatographed on Amberlite CG-50 (H+) and silica gel, to eliminate free amino acids and nonpolar dyes.

RESULTS

Chromatography of the heat-treated cell sap on CM-cellulose

The 55 ml of rat liver cell sap were treated at 55° for exactly 3 min under gentle agitation and then cooled in ice water. Precipitates were centrifuged down and washed 3 times with an equal volume of 0.01 M Tris–HCl buffer (pH 7.0). The supernatants were combined. Protein, protein-bound dye and arginase, assayed before and after the heat treatment of the cell sap, showed that more than 70% of the cell sap proteins were removed as insoluble precipitates after the heat treatment, while both azo dye-binding protein and arginase activity were retained almost completely in the supernatant. This simple procedure increased the specific dye-binding as well as the specific arginase activity of the cell sap almost 10-fold with satisfactory yields. The procedure seemed to be useful because a large part of the heme proteins that interfere with the accurate assay of protein-bound dye was removed.

The heat-treated rat liver cell sap was dialysed against 0.01 M Tris–HCl buffer (pH 7.0) overnight, and an aliquot of the dialysate was subjected to chromatography on CM-cellulose. The elution pattern of proteins, as well as arginase activity, is illustrated in Fig. 1. The distribution of protein, protein-bound dye and arginase among fractionated protein groups is summarized in Table I.

As shown in Fig. 1, the largest protein band was observed in the preliminary eluate (Fraction I), a small protein band in the 0.01-M NaCl eluate, the second largest protein band in the 0.02-M NaCl (Fraction IV), and two small bands in the 0.05-M NaCl (Fractions VI and VII) eluates. As shown in Table I, protein-bound dye was mainly located in Fractions I (40–50%), IV (11–15%), VI (2.4%) and VII (4.0%). On the other hand, the arginase activity was detected mainly in Fractions VI (35%) and VII (33%) though activity was also found in Fractions I (15%) and IV (19%), suggesting a polymorphic nature of rat liver arginase[15]. In another experimental run,

163

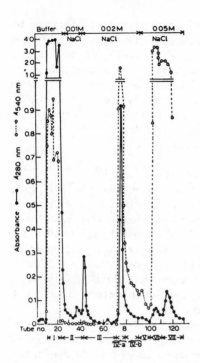

Fig. 1. Elution pattern of the heat-treated (55°, 3 min) rat liver cell sap proteins subjected to chromatography on CM-cellulose (40 h, 3'-MDAB). Starting from 55 ml of the 50% liver cell sap prepared 40 h after administration of 40 mg of 3'-MDAB, 166 ml of the heat-treated cell sap (combined with washings of the denatured protein precipitates) were obtained. A 66-ml portion was applied to a CM-cellulose column (2 cm × 26 cm). Stepwise elution was carried out by running 0.01 M Tris–HCl buffer (pH 7.0), 0.01, 0.02 and 0.05 M NaCl in the same buffer successively. ●—●, A_{280} nm as a rough estimate of proteins; ○—○ arginase activity as expressed by A_{520} nm at the assay of generated urea according to the method of VAN SLYKE AND ARCHIBALD[13].

TABLE I

DISTRIBUTION OF PROTEINS, PROTEIN-BOUND DYE AND ARGINASE OF THE HEAT-TREATED RAT LIVER CELL SAP AMONG FRACTION GROUPS SEPARATED BY CHROMATOGRAPHY ON CM-CELLULOSE 40 h, 3'-MDAB.

Fraction group	Tube No.	Protein (%)	Protein-bound dye (%)	Arginase (%)	Bound dye (nmoles/mg protein)	Arginase (units per mg protein)
Cell sap		1600	117	96	0.19	0.46
Heated cell sap		100	100	100	2.66	7.60
I	10–22	57.5	41.0	15	1.42	1.01
II	23–42	15.5	6.7	—	0.86	—
III	43–71	3.7	—	—	—	—
IV-a	72–77	3.9	11.1	19(a+b)	5.60	7.0(a+b)
IV-b	78–90	4.5	3.5		1.57	
V	91–99	1.6	—	—	—	—
VI	100–110	3.1	2.4	35	1.58	43.7
VII	111–126	4.5	4.0	33	1.78	27.6
Sum	10–126	94.6	69.0	102	2.00	7.6

the rat liver cell sap without the heat treatment (55°, 3 min) was subjected to chromatography in the same way. The arginase activity was, however, mainly found in Fraction 1 (52%) and the percentages of arginase present in Fractions IV, VI and VII were 10, 16 and 21%, respectively. Therefore the apparent polymorphic behaviour of the rat liver arginase might be partly due to some interactions of arginase with other components. Heat treatment of the liver cell sap seems largely to eliminate the interacting components as denatured precipitates. In contrast with that of arginase, the distribution pattern of dye-bound proteins was similar regardless of the heat treatment (Fraction I > Fraction IV > Fraction VII > Fraction VI).

Further purification of dye-binding proteins in Fractions I, IV and VII

When Fraction I was subjected to differential precipitation with $(NH_4)_2SO_4$, 70% of the protein-bound dye was recovered in the 100% saturation precipitate while 30% remained in the supernatant. The precipitated proteins were immediately dissolved in 0.01 M Tris buffer (pH 7.0) and dialysed against the same buffer. The 100% saturation supernatant was dialysed against the same Tris buffer and the dialysate was concentrated with the aid of a collodion filter. A 3-ml portion of each 100% saturation precipitate (Fraction I-100(ppt.)) and supernatant (Fraction I-100(sup.)) was subjected to gel filtration on Sephadex G-100. The elution patterns of Fraction I-100(ppt.) and Fraction I-100(sup.) are illustrated in Fig. 2.

From Fraction I-100 (ppt.) almost 90% of the protein-bound dye was recovered in the first band (Band 1), while from Fraction I-100 (sup.) most of the protein-bound dye was found in the last band (Band 5). These results indicate that the dye-binding proteins in Fraction I consisted of at least two molecular species, one high-molecular-weight protein and another low-molecular-weight one.

In another experimental run starting from 100 ml of Fraction I (0.91 mg protein per ml) the pH of the solution was lowered stepwise by the addition of 1 M acetic acid to pH 5.5, 5.0 and 4.0 under cooling in ice. Considerable precipitates were generated at pH 5.5 and 5.0, but no more precipitation occurred below pH 5.0. The precipitates

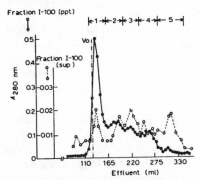

Fig. 2. Gel filtration of $(NH_4)_2SO_4$ 100% satn. precipitate (Fraction I-100 (ppt.)) and supernatant (Fraction I-100 (sup.)) fractions from Fraction I. 3 ml each of the Fraction I-100(ppt.) dialysate and the concentrated Fraction I-100 (sup.) dialysate were applied to a Sephadex G-100 column (2.8 cm × 62 cm). The elution was carried out by running 0.1 M KCl in 0.05 M Tris–HCl buffer (pH 7.5). Protein-bound dye was found mainly in the first band (1) of Fraction I-100 (ppt.) and mainly in the last band (5) of Fraction I-100 (sup.).

165

at pH 5.5 and 5.0 were immediately suspended in 0.01 M Tris–HCl buffer (pH 7.0), and the proteins were dissolved by the addition of 1 M Tris base. The pH 5.0 supernatant was also neutralized by means of 1 M Tris base. Proteins recovered in the pH 5.5 precipitate, the pH 5.0 precipitate and the pH 5.0 supernatant were 20, 7 and 75%, respectively, while protein-bound dye recovered in these fractions were 21, 9 and 62%.

The pH 5.0 supernatant (Fraction I-pH 5.0 (sup.)) neutralized with Tris base was then dialysed against 0.01 M Tris–HCl buffer (pH 7.0), followed by concentration by collodion filtration. 2 ml of the concentrated sample (protein 18.7 mg and protein-bound dye 18 nmoles) were subjected to gel filtration in the same way. The elution pattern of Fraction I-pH 5.0 (sup.) proteins was similar to that of Fraction I-100 (ppt.) except that it had a higher peak 5. The percentages of proteins in Peaks 1, 2, 3 + 4 and 5 were 21, 7, 39 and 9%, respectively, while the protein-bound dye in Peak 1 was 19% and that in Peak 5 was 50%.

These results indicate that the low-molecular-weight dye-binding protein in Fraction I was enriched in the pH 5.0 supernatant (Fraction I-pH 5 (sup.)), while the high-molecular-weight dye-binding protein was enriched in the $(NH_4)_2SO_4$ 100% saturation precipitate (Fraction I-100 (ppt.)).

The two dye-bound proteins thus isolated from Fraction I (Fraction I-100 (ppt.)-1 and Fraction I-pH 5.0 (sup.)-5) showed specific dye-binding of 7.8 and 5.7 nmoles dye per mg protein, repectively. If we adopt the molecular weights of 170 000 and 12 000 for these proteins, respectively, as calculated from the elution volumes. the specific dye-binding in terms of dye mole per mole protein becomes 1.3 for the high-molecular-weight dye-binding protein (I-a) and 0.07 for the low-molecular-weight dye-binding protein (I-b).

Purification of the dye-binding protein in Fraction IV was carried out similarly. The dye-bound protein in Fraction IV was precipitated completely by $(NH_4)_2SO_4$ at 60% saturation. The precipitate (Fraction IV-60 (ppt.)) was dissolved in 0.01 M Tris–HCl buffer (pH 7.0) and dialysed against the same buffer. A 3-ml aliquot of the dialysate was subjected to gel filtration on Sephadex G-100. As illustrated in Fig. 3a, the elution pattern indicates one major and two minor protein bands (in terms of $A_{280\ nm}$) or two major chromoprotein bands (in terms of $A'_{410\ nm}$). The first chromoprotein band (Fraction IV-60 (ppt.)-1) was located in the front half of the first major protein band, and the second chromoprotein band corresponded to the last minor protein band (Fraction IV-60 (ppt.)-3). The assay of protein-bound dye, however, revealed that only the first chromoprotein band contained aminoazo dye bound to protein and thus the last chromoprotein seemed to be heme-containing. The arginase activity in Fraction IV was mainly recovered in a protein fraction between the two chromoprotein bands (Fraction IV-60 (ppt.)-2).

Since the amount of dye-bound protein in Fraction VII was rather small, Fraction VII was directly dialysed against 0.01 M Tris–HCl buffer (pH 7.0) without differential precipitation, and the dialysate was concentrated by collodion filtration. A 3-ml aliquot of the concentrated. Fraction VII was subjected to gel filtration as above. The elution pattern, as illustrated in Fig. 3b, indicates three chromoprotein peaks (1, 2 and 3). The protein-bound dye was distributed as follows: 43% in Peak 1, 21% in Peak 2 and 39% in Peak 3. The extraordinarily high absorbance at 410 nm of Peak 3 seemed to be due to the copresence of heme protein(s).

Specific dye bindings of Fractions IV-60 (ppt.)-1 (IV), VII-1 (VII-a) and VII-3

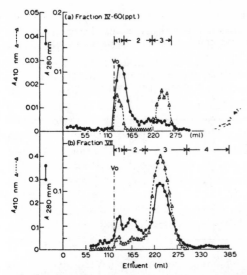

Fig. 3. Gel filtration of $(NH_4)_2SO_4$ 60% satn. precipitate from Fraction IV and of Fraction VII. The $(NH_4)_2SO_4$ 60% satn. precipitate of Fraction IV was dissolved in a small volume of 0.01 M Tris–HCl buffer (pH 7.0) and dialysed against the same buffer. Fraction VII was directly dialysed against the same buffer and concentrated by collodion filtration. A 3-ml aliquot from each sample was applied to a Sephadex G-100 column (2.8 cm × 62 cm), and elution was carried out as described in METHODS AND MATERIALS. "a" indicates the elution pattern of Fraction IV proteins and "b" that of Fraction VII proteins. Most of the protein-bound dye was detected in the first peak (68%) of Fraction IV while protein-bound dye was detected in the first chromoprotein peak (43%) and the third peak (39%) of Fraction VII.

(VII-b) were 9.0, 6.0 and 0.18 nmoles dye per mg protein. If we adopt the molecular weights of 160 000, 160 000 and 40 000 for IV, VII-a and VII-b dye-binding proteins, the specific dye bindings, as expressed in terms of mole dye per mole protein, become 1.4, 1.0 and 0.01, respectively.

As stated above, most (nearly 70%) of the arginase activity in the heat-treated liver cell sap was recovered in the basic protein fractions (Fractions VI and VII). In gel filtration of Fraction VII, the arginase activity was mainly (82%) recovered in the second peak (Fraction VII-2) corresponding to the molecular weight of 130 000.

Electrophoresis of some of the separated dye-binding proteins

The electrophoresis of Fractions I-100 (ppt.), IV-60 (ppt.) and VII in the veronal buffer (pH 8.6) showed 5, 3 and 4–5 protein bands, respectively, in accordance with the heterogeneity revealed by the gel-filtration results as described above. With Fraction I-100 (ppt.) the protein-bound dye was detected in the two fast-moving bands, while with Fractions IV-60 (ppt.) and VII the protein-bound dye was detected in only one band moving only slightly to the anodic side (Fraction IV-60) or completely immobile (Fraction VII).

The electrophoretograms of Fractions I-100 (ppt.)-1 (I-a), IV-60 (ppt.)-1 (IV) and VII-1 (VII-a) indicated only two protein bands. In each electrophoretogram protein-bound dye was detected only in a major protein component. The dependence of electrophoretic mobility upon pH of dye-bound proteins in Fig. 4 shows isoelectric

167

TABLE II

DISTRIBUTION OF PROTEINS, PROTEIN-BOUND DYE AND ARGINASE OF THE HEAT-TREATED RAT LIVER CELL SAP AMONG FRACTION GROUPS SEPARATED BY CHROMATOGRAPHY ON CM-CELLULOSE 40 h, 2-MDAB.

Fraction group	Protein (%)	Protein-bound dye (%)	Arginase (%)	Bound dye (nmoles/mg protein)	Arginase (units/mg protein)
Cell sap	1500	94	123	0.07	0.34
Heated cell sap	100	100	100	1.14	4.06
I	63	5.8	1.4	0.1	0.09
II	11.5	2.0	0.2	0.2	0.08
III	6	—	0.1	—	0.08
IV-a	9.8	52.8	3.8	6.1	1.60
IV-b	4.8	13.8	3.4	3.2	2.85
V	3.8	—	3.8	—	4.14
VI	2.8	6.0	28.0	2.4	40.0
VII	5.1	7.1	28.5	1.6	27.7
Sum	107	87.7	69.5		

points of 5.2 for I-a and 8.0 for IV dye-binding proteins. Since VII-a dye-binding protein did not migrate at pH 8.6, its isoelectric point seemed to be near pH 8.6. Apparently the dye-binding proteins in the rat liver cell sap were different from the dye-binding protein (albumin) in the serum, at least electrophoretically.

Protein-binding pattern of 2-MDAB

The rat liver cell sap was prepared 40 h after administration of 40 mg of 2-MDAB. The 15 ml of liver cell sap thus prepared was treated at 55° for 3 min, and the supernatant combined with washings of the precipitates was dialysed against 0.01 M Tris–HCl buffer (pH 7.0). An aliquot of the dialysate was subjected to chromatography on CM-cellulose. The elution pattern of proteins as expressed in terms of A_{280} nm was similar to that of the normal liver cell sap or liver cell sap from rats given 3′-MDAB

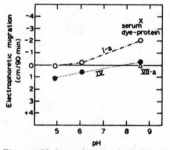

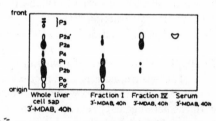

Fig. 4. pH-dependence of electrophoretic mobility of dye-bound proteins. The conditions of electrophoresis are described in METHODS AND MATERIALS. ○—·—○, Fraction I-100 (ppt.)-1 dye-binding protein (I-a); ●·····●, Fraction IV-60 (ppt.)-1 dye binding protein(IV); △, Fraction VII-1 dye-binding protein (VII-a); X, dye-binding protein in the rat serum.

Fig. 5. Chromatogram of the polar dyes, prepared from the whole liver cell sap, Fraction I, Fraction IV and the serum, on cellulose thin-layer plates. The polar dyes were prepared by a large excess of pronase or repeated pronase treatment, spotted onto cellulose thin-layer plates (10 cm × 10 cm) and developed in an aqueous phase from a mixture of n-propanol–n-butanol–water (1:4:5, by vol.) (ascending). After development the plates were exposed to HCl fumes over conc. HCl.

(Fig. 1). The assay of protein-bound dye, however, revealed an entirely different feature. As summarized in Table II, the percentages of proteins in Fractions I, IV, VI and VII were 63, 14, 2.8 and 5.1, respectively, while protein-bound dye in these fractional groups was 6, 67, 6 and 7%, respectively.

The facts that noncarcinogenic (or, more strictly, very weakly carcinogenic) 2-MDAB is bound to Fraction IV preferentially and that the binding to Fraction I is very small seem to suggest that the dye-binding to Fraction IV may not be relevant to the carcinogenic mechanism.

Nature of polar dyes prepared from Fractions I and IV separated from the liver cell sap of rats given 3'-MDAB

The polar dyes prepared from Fraction I and IV and from the whole rat liver cell sap were subjected to thin-layer chromatography on cellulose, using an aqueous phase from a mixture of n-propanol–n-butanol–water (1:4:5, by vol.) or a mixture of acetone–water (1:3, v/v) as the solvent. The chromatograms of the polar dye components thus obtained are illustrated in Fig. 5.

Fraction I gave polar dye components similar to those from the whole liver cell sap, *i.e.* P2b and P1 as major components in addition to P2a and P2a', whereas the polar dye prepared from Fraction IV gave only P2a and P2a' and lacked P2b and P1 which have been reported to be methionine-derived polar dyes[16,17]. P2a (and probably P2a') is considered to be tyrosine derived[18,19].

TABLE III

ISOLATED DYE-BINDING PROTEINS AND THEIR CHARACTERISTICS (FROM THE LIVER CELL SAP OF RATS) 40 H AFTER THE ADMINISTRATION OF 40 MG OF 3'-MDAB.

The approximate concentration of dye-binding protein was calculated at the purification stage of Sephadex gel filtration. Usually at this stage of purification, another protein band in addition to dye-bound protein could be detected on electrophoretograms. Therefore, actual concentrations should be less than the values listed above. The order of abundance in the liver cell sap was I-b>I-a>VII-b>IV>VII-a, while I-a ≈ IV>VII-a>I-b>VII-b in the order of degree of modification.

Nomenclature of protein	Electrolytic nature (isoelectric point)	Mol. wt.	Specific dye binding (mole dye/mole protein)	Approximate concn. (% of total cell sap proteins)
I-a	Non-basic (5.2)	160 000–170 000	1.3	<0.5
I-b	Non-basic	12 000–15 000	0.07	<0.7
IV	Slightly basic (8.0)	160 000–170 000	1.4	<0.05
VII-a	More basic (8.6)	160 000–170 000	1.0	<0.01
VII-b	More basic	40 000	0.01	<0.2

Dye-binding protein in rat serum prepared 40 h after administration of 3'-MDAB

The serum was prepared from the blood of rats killed 40 h after administration of a single large dose (40 mg) of 3'-MDAB. The serum diluted 5-fold with 0.01 M Tris–HCl buffer (pH 7.0) was dialysed against the same buffer, and the dialysate was subjected to chromatography on CM-cellulose as described above.

An elution pattern similar to that of the rat liver cell sap was observed, but protein-bound dye was found predominantly in the preliminary eluate (90%). Only a small portion (each 2.6%) was found in the basic fractions analogous to Fractions VI and VII, and the binding to a fraction analogous to Fraction IV was negligibly

169

small. 40 ml of the preliminary eluate were dialysed against 0.01 M Tris–HCl buffer (pH 6.5) and the dialysate was applied to a DEAE-Sephadex (A-50) column (1.5 cm × 16 cm). After the column had been washed with the buffer, stepwise elution was carried out by running 0.05, 0.1 and 0.25 M NaCl in the same buffer, successively. The protein-bound dye was found predominantly in a fraction eluted by 0.1 M NaCl. Since the serum albumin has been confirmed to be eluted in this fraction, the present results support previous reports that the carcinogenic aminoazo dye can bind to serum albumin[20,21]. The polar dye prepared from the serum gave only P2a'.

DISCUSSION

This paper describes the isolation of carcinogenic aminoazo dye-bound proteins from the liver of rats killed 40 h after the administration of a single large dose (40 mg) of 3'-MDAB. In parallel with the present study we have undertaken the isolation of dye-binding proteins from the liver of rats fed the 3'-MDAB-containing diet continuously for certain periods and the results will soon be published.

It has been reported that the amount of protein-bound dye is similar no matter how the carcinogenic aminoazo dye is administered, *i.e.* single large-dose administration or continuous feeding, so long as the protein-bound dye is measured at the time of maximal binding. This peak in the dye-protein binding is reached 40 h after intragastric administration of a large dose (40 mg) of 3'-MDAB and after 2–3 weeks of continuous feeding of 0.06% 3'-MDAB diet. However, no systematic study has been reported concerning the nature of dye-binding proteins under the two experimental conditions.

Using the liver of rats continuously fed the 3'-MDAB-containing diet, SOROF et al.[9] reported that the major dye-binding protein in the rat liver cell sap is a basic protein belonging to the slow h_2 fraction and having the molecular weight of 60 000–80 000. KETTERER et al.[10] purified the basic dye-binding protein of molecular weight of 45 000 in the liver cell sap of rats given a single large dose of 3'-MDAB. The two groups have reported the presence of dye-binding proteins of low molecular weight of 10 000–15 000 in addition to the major dye-binding proteins of basic nature. The presence of dye-binding proteins having the molecular weight of 40 000 (VII-b) as well as 12 000–15 000 (I-b) has been confirmed in the present study. Sorof's dye-binding protein having the molecular weight of 60 000–80 000, however, could not be detected in the present study. It might be present in Fraction VI which has not yet been investigated because of the scarcity of the sample. However, this possibility seems to be small, mainly for the following reasons.

As will be reported in another paper (in preparation) a basic dye-binding protein having the molecular weight of 68 000 has been isolated from the liver of rats continuously fed the 3'-MDAB diet for 1 month, supporting the results of SOROF et al.[9]. This dye-binding protein was eluted in a band behind Fraction VII in the chromatography on CM-cellulose. The band as such is absent or negligibly small in the liver cell sap shortly after 3'-MDAB administration.

In the present paper a few new dye-binding proteins having the molecular weight of 160 000–170 000 have been isolated. They were found in Fractions I (I-a), IV (IV) and VII (VII-a).

I-a dye-binding protein is apparently nonbasic and seems to have an isoelectric point of 5.2. It should be emphasized that I-a is the major target protein in the normal liver cell sap. The reason why KETTERER *et al.* failed to find this protein seems to be as follows. They eliminated almost two-thirds of the dye-bound proteins in the rat liver cell sap by precipitation at pH 4.5 in the presence of Cu^{2+}, Ca^{2+} and NaCl before proceeding to chromatographic isolation of the basic dye-binding protein. This procedure may be useful for the isolation of the basic dye-binding protein of molecular weight of 45 000, but seemingly they lost the major dye-binding protein of nonbasic nature and at the same time some basic dye-binding proteins of high molecular weight.

The dye-binding protein in Fraction IV is slightly basic (isoelectric point near 8) and has the high molecular weight of 160 000–170 000. This dye-binding protein, however, seems to be of less significance mainly because almost noncarcinogenic 2-MDAB is bound primarily to this protein. The more basic dye-binding proteins which have been found in Fraction VII seem to consist of at least two components; one has the molecular weight of 160 000–170 000 (VII-a) and another has the molecular weight of 40 000 (VII-b). Under the present experimental conditions, the specific dye-binding of VII-a was 1.0 mole dye per mole protein while that of VII-b was only 0.01 mole dye per mole protein, although the abundance of VII-a in the cell sap (less than 0.01%) was much smaller than that of VII-b (less than 0.2%). For this reason VII-a dye-binding protein seems to be more essential for the molecular mechanism of carcinogenesis. A similar discussion would also be applicable to the dye-binding proteins in Fraction I. I-a and I-b are present in the liver cell sap in almost equal concentration (less than 0.5–0.7%). However, I-a, having the molecular weight of 160 000–170 000, can be modified with the dye almost entirely (1.3 mole dye per mole protein), whereas I-b, having the molecular weight of 12 000–15 000, is modified only slightly (0.07 mole dye per mole protein).

The reason why SOROF *et al.*[7–9] did not find the dye-binding proteins of high molecular weight, such as I-a, IV and VII-a, seems to be that they used the liver cell sap of rats fed the 3'-MDAB diet for 18–20 days. A parallel study (in preparation) has shown that these dye-binding proteins are deleted soon after the onset of dye-feeding, and to our great interest are replaced by new dye-binding proteins of more and more basic nature. Thus, the dye-binding proteins in the liver cell sap of rats fed 3'-MDAB for a few weeks consist primarily of the more basic proteins which are eluted behind Fraction VII.

In the present study it has been elucidated that the amino acid residue involved in the binding to azo dye is rather specific to the nature of the receptor protein. For example, the polar dye prepared from Fraction I gave P2b and P1 as the major polar dye components, while the polar dye from Fraction IV or the serum gave P2a and P2a' as the major components. Investigations on the polar dyes from other dye-binding proteins are now in progress.

As to the identity of rat liver arginase with the dye-binding proteins, the results of the present study seem to be rather negative. The dye-binding proteins in both Fractions IV and VII were well separated from the arginase activity in the Sephadex gel filtration.

ACKNOWLEDGEMENTS

The authors wish to express their thanks to Dr. M. Matsumoto for valuable

171

discussions and advice throughout the present study. A part of the expenses for the present study was covered by the Grant-in-Aid for Scientific Research from the Ministry of Education.

REFERENCES

1 E. C. MILLER AND J. A. MILLER, Cancer Res., 7 (1947) 468.
2 E. C. MILLER AND J. A. MILLER, Cancer Res., 12 (1952) 547.
3 E. K. WEISBURGER, J. H. WEISBURGER AND H. P. MORRIS, Arch. Biochem. Biophys., 43 (1953) 474.
4 E. C. MILLER, Cancer Res., 10 (1950) 232.
5 W. G. WIEST AND C. HEIDELBERGER, Cancer Res., 13 (1953) 250.
6 S. SOROF, P. P. COHEN, E. C. MILLER AND J. A. MILLER, Cancer Res., 11 (1951) 383.
7 S. SOROF, E. M. YOUNG, M. M. McCUE AND P. L. FETTERMAN, Cancer Res., 23 (1963) 864.
8 S. SOROF, E. M. YOUNG, L. LUONGS, V. KISH AND J. J. FREED, Wistar Symp. Monograph, 7 (1967) 25.
9 S. SOROF, Jerusalem Symp. Quantum Chem. Biol. Chem., 1 (1969) 208.
10 B. KETTERER, P. ROSS-MANSELL AND J. K. WHITEHEAD, Biochem. J., 103 (1967) 316.
11 G. WARWICK, European J. Cancer, 3 (1967) 227.
12 O. H. LOWRY, N. J. ROSEBROUGH, A. L. FARR AND R. T. RANDALL, J. Biol. Chem., 193 (1951) 265.
13 D. D. VAN SLYKE AND R. M. ARCHIBALD, J. Biol. Chem., 165 (1946) 293.
14 H. TERAYAMA, in H. BUSCH, Methods in Cancer Research, Vol. 1, Academic Press, New York, 1967, p. 339.
15 S. SOROF AND V. M. KISH, Cancer Res., 29 (1969) 261.
16 T. HIGASHINAKAGAWA, M. MATSUMOTO AND H. TERAYAMA, Biochem. Biophys. Res. Commun., 24 (1966) 811.
17 J.-K. LIN, J. A. MILLER AND E. C. MILLER, Biochemistry, 7 (1968) 1889.
18 J.-K. LIN, J. A. MILLER AND E. C. MILLER, Biochemistry, 8 (1969) 1573.
19 M. MATSUMOTO AND H. TERAYAMA, Chem.-Biol. Interactions, 1 (1969/70) 73.
20 K. KUSAMA, Nippon Kagaku Zasshi, 81 (1960) 763.
21 J. DIJKSTRA AND H. M. GRIGGS, Proc. IXth Intern. Cancer Congr., (1966) 183.

Partial Purification of Soluble Protein from Mouse Skin to Which Carcinogenic Hydrocarbons Are Specifically Bound

Judith G. Tasseron, Heino Diringer, Nechama Frohwirth,

S. S. Mirvish, and Charles Heidelberger

Following the initial demonstration by Miller (1951) of the binding of carcinogenic hydrocarbons to mouse epidermal proteins using fluorescent techniques, a study of this phenomenon has continued in this laboratory by means of tracer methodology. Wiest and Heidelberger (1953) established the covalent nature of this interaction in the case 1,2,5,6-DBA,[1] and a rough correlation between the binding to total mouse skin proteins of various polycyclic aromatic hydrocarbons and their carcinogenic activity was demonstrated by Heidel-

---

[1] Abbreviations used are: DBA, dibenzanthracene; MCA, methylcholanthrene.

berger and Moldenhauer (1956). On preliminary fractionation of the proteins of mouse skin, the hydrocarbons did not appear to be bound to any specific fraction (Davenport *et al.*, 1961). However, Abell and Heidelberger (1962) carried out starch gel electrophoresis of the soluble proteins of mouse skin following topical application of tritiated hydrocarbons and found a radioactive band with covalently bound carcinogens. They described the striking correlation between the binding to this protein fraction and the carcinogenic process; hence, it was of obvious interest to attempt to purify, isolate, and characterize this protein from mouse skin.

The partial purification of the rat liver protein to which the azo dyes and acetylaminofluorene are bound has been accomplished by Sorof and his colleagues (*cf*. 1963), using vertical column electrophoresis. He has termed this the h_2 fraction. His more recent work has been reviewed (Sorof, 1969). Barry and Gutmann (1966) have also partially purified the rat liver protein to which acetylaminofluorene is bound, by chromatography on Sephadex G-25 and DEAE-cellulose. Apparently the most complete purification of this rat liver protein to date has been accomplished by Ketterer *et al.* (1967). However, the identity of this as the main protein to which the azo dyes are bound has been questioned by Sorof (1969). Since the protein in mouse skin to which the hydrocarbons are bound in quantitative relationship to their carcinogenic activities has some properties similar to the *h* protein of Sorof, we will henceforth refer to this as the mouse skin *h* protein.

Materials and Methods

Animals. Female Swiss albino mice weighing 25–30 g, obtained from the A. R. Schmidt Co., Madison, Wis., were used. They were fed Rockland pellets and water *ad libitum.*

Chemicals. Tritiated 1,2,5,6-DBA, 1,2,3,4-DBA, and 3-MCA were obtained from Amersham-Searle. They were diluted with the corresponding nonradioactive hydrocarbons obtained from Eastman Organic Chemicals to a suitable final specific activity, in most cases 100 mCi/mmol. The radiochemical purity of the hydrocarbons was periodically checked by thin-layer chromatography, and only homogeneous samples were used.

The following proteins were used for the molecular weight determinations: ovalbumin from the Nutritional Biochemicals

174

Corp., horse heart cytochrome c and papain from the Sigma Chemical Corp., deoxyribonuclease I and elastase from Worthington Biochemical Corp., transferrin from Behringwerke, bovine serum albumin from Pentex Inc., and bromgrass mosaic virus.

Measurements of Radioactivity. Radioactivity was measured in a Packard Tri-Carb liquid scintillation spectrometer. Aqueous solutions were counted in Scintisol (Isolab, Inc.).

Radioactivity was measured in protein precipitates by dissolving them in 1 ml of Soluene (Packard Instrument Co.) to which 10 ml of toluene–2,5-diphenyloxazole (Liquifluor, New England Nuclear Corp.) was added.

Slices of stained polyacrylamide gels were incubated with 0.5 ml of Soluene in capped counting vials at 50° overnight. This procedure made the pieces swell considerably and eluted the protein from the gel. After addition of 10 ml of toluene–2,5-diphenyloxazole the slices were counted. This method gives a higher counting efficiency than digestion of the gel slices by the hydrogen peroxide method of Young and Fulhorst (1965).

Preparation of the Skin Protein Extract. ^{3}H-Labeled hydrocarbon (0.1 mg in 0.1 ml of benzene/mouse, 100 mCi/mmol) was dropped on the backs of 100 mice, which had been clipped the previous day. After 48 hr, when maximum binding occurs (Abell and Heidelberger, 1962) the mice were killed with ether. The skins of the backs were dissected and the adipose tissue and blood vessels were removed by scraping the inside of the skin with razor blades. The skins were frozen in liquid nitrogen immediately. The frozen skins were pulverized inside four thicknesses of cheesecloth with a wooden mallet and homogenized in 170 ml of 0.01 M Tris-HCl buffer (pH 8.0), containing 0.01 M NaCl, with a Polytron (Type PT 10 O.D. Kinematica GMBA, Luzern, Switzerland). The homogenate was centrifuged at 100,000g for 1 hr and the pink supernatant was filtered through glass wool to remove the layer of fat.

Purification of the Mouse Skin h Protein. All purification steps were performed at 4° in a cold room.

STEP 1. SEPARATION OF THE LOW AND HIGH MOLECULAR WEIGHT SUBSTANCES. The high-speed supernatant fraction (175 ml from 100 mice) was passed through a Sephadex G-25 column (6.5 × 40 cm) with the same 0.01 M Tris-HCl buffer (pH 8.0) containing 0.01 M NaCl used for the extraction. The high molecular weight fraction was well separated from the low molecular weight material and was collected in fractions 10–26, each tube containing 16 ml. Elution of the low molecular weight material started at about fraction 28. The

175

radioactivity in this latter fraction trailed over a big volume, which was found with all hydrocarbons. The adsorption of low molecular weight aromatic compounds to Sephadex is well known (*cf.* Determann and Walter, 1968).

STEP 2. DEAE-CELLULOSE CHROMATOGRAPHY. The Sephadex G-25 high molecular weight fraction (about 250 ml) was immediately passed through a DEAE-cellulose column (Serva, 0.7 mequiv/g, 15 g/100 skins, column 3.5 × 7 cm) in the same buffer as used for Sephadex G-25 fractionation. The least acidic proteins passed through the column without retention. This fraction was concentrated to 20–30 ml according to the method of Blatt *et al.* (1965) by ultrafiltration through a Diaflo UM10 membrane (Amicon Corp.), which retains substances of molecular weight greater than 10,000. Further concentration to 2–3 ml was achieved by reverse dialysis with Ficoll powder (Pharmacia). During these concentration procedures the small amount of precipitate that formed was checked for radioactivity, which was invariably low, and it was discarded.

STEP 3. SEPHADEX G-100 GEL FILTRATION. The concentrated DEAE-cellulose breakthrough peak was carefully layered on top of a Sephadex G-100 column (2.5 × 140 cm). The column was developed with 0.01 M Tris-HCl buffer (pH 8.0), containing 0.01 M NaCl and 0.005 M β-mercaptoethanol at a flow rate of approximately 15 ml/hr. Fractions of 8 ml were collected. The radioactive peak was concentrated by dialysis against Ficoll. The concentrated fraction was stored frozen after addition of one-tenth volume glycerol or was used fresh for the isoelectric focusing procedure. Repeated freezing and thawing did not affect the proteins, as shown on Sephadex G-100 and by isoelectric focusing in polyacrylamide gels, which gave the same patterns as the fresh unfrozen solution.

STEP 4. ISOELECTRIC FOCUSING PROCEDURE. The method described by Vesterberg and Svensson (1966) was used. The isoelectric focusing was performed in an LKB8100 electrofocusing column. The pH gradient used was either from pH 6 to 9 or from pH 7 to 9. These gradients were obtained with carrier ampholytes (LKB Instruments, Inc.). The anode was placed at the top of the column, the cathode at the bottom. Between the electrode solutions a sucrose density gradient containing 1% carrier ampholytes was arranged to prevent convection during the separation. The gradient was prepared in 24 tubes containing 4.6 ml of a mixture of systematically varied amounts of a 50% sucrose solution containing 1.5% ampholytes and a less dense solution (without sucrose) containing 0.5% ampholytes. The first tube contained 4.6 ml of the dense solution, the second contained 4.4 ml of dense solution and 0.2 ml of less dense solution, and so on. The radioactive *h* protein fraction eluted from the Sephadex G-100 column replaced the less dense solutions in the 11–13 tubes, after dialysis overnight against 1% amphclytes. The contents of the individual tubes were well mixed before they were successively poured down the glass wall into the column: the most dense solution was added first.

The column was run for 3 days and was cooled with water circulated at 4°. The voltage applied at first was 300 V, which was increased to 500 V after 24 hr and 600 V after 48 hr. After the run, fractions of 36 drops were collected. The pH of the fractions was measured with a Radiometer pH meter, Model PHM26. The fractions were assayed for radioactivity and optical density at 260 and 280 mμ. The radioactive fractions in the pH 8.05 region were concentrated by dialysis against Ficoll and kept frozen after addition of a 10% volume of glycerol for further testing. Replicate runs were highly reproducible.

Disc electrophoresis was carried out in the equipment made by Canalco, Rockville, Md. Three different types of electrophoresis were used.

BASIC SYSTEM, 7% POLYACRYLAMIDE GEL. The polymerization solution contained volumes of solutions A–B–C–H$_2$O of 1:2:4:1. Solution A contained 36.3 g of Tris, 48 ml of 1 N HCl, 0.23 ml of N,N,N,N'-tetramethylethylenediamine, and H$_2$O to 100 ml. Solution B contained 28.0 g of acrylamide, 0.735 g of N,N'-methylenebisacrylamide, and H$_2$O to 100 ml. Solution C (always freshly made) contained 0.14 g of ammonium persulfate in 100 ml of H$_2$O. The gels were 5.5 mm wide and 6 cm high. The tray buffer solution contained 0.0248 M Tris and 0.192 M glycine per l. (pH 8.3). The run was performed at 4° and at 4 mA/gel. The gels were fixed and stained in an Amido Black solution in 7.5% acetic acid and destained by repeated washing in 7.5% acetic acid.

BASIC SYSTEM, DIFFERENT POLYACRYLAMIDE GEL CONCENTRATIONS. A variation of the first method was used for the estimation of molecular weight (Hedrick and Smith, 1968). Solution B contained 24 g of acrylamide and 0.8 g of $N\,N'$-methylenebisacrylamide. By proper dilutions gels were made containing 5, 7, 9, and 11% acrylamide. The molecular weight of proteins can be calculated from the slope of the graph where 100 log ($R_m \times 100$) is plotted against the gel concentration, where R_m is the mobility relative to bromophenol blue.

SODIUM DODECYL SULFATE–POLYACRYLAMIDE GEL SYSTEM. A modification of the system described by Shapiro *et al.* (1967) was used. The gels contained 0.1% sodium dodecyl sulfate, 0.1 M Tris (pH 7.3), 7% acrylamide, 0.4% N,N'-methylene-

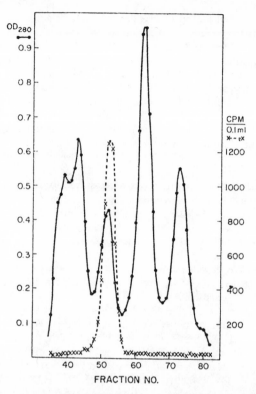

FIGURE 1: Sephadex G-100 gel filtration of the breakthrough peak from a DEAE-cellulose column. The fractions contained 7 ml. The buffer was 0.01 M Tris-HCl (pH 8.0) containing 0.01 M NaCl and 0.005 M β-mercaptoethanol. The mice had been treated with MCA.

bisacrylamide, and 8 M urea. The tray buffer contained 0.1 M Tris (pH 7.3), 8 M urea, 0.1% sodium dodecyl sulfate, and 0.1% 2-aminoethanethiol hydrochloride. This buffer was used in the bottom electrode bath. The same buffer without urea was used in the top electrode bath. The sample contained 50 μg of protein in 0.1 M Tris (pH 7.3), 8 M urea, 1% sodium dodecyl sulfate, and 0.1% 2-aminoethanethiol hydrochloride. The electrophoresis was carried out at room temperature at 7 mA/gel. The gels were fixed in 10% acetic acid, 50% methanol, and 40% H₂O for 2 hr, stained in 20% methanol, 0.5% Amido Black, and 2.2% acetic acid for 2 hr and destained by repeated washing with 35% ethanol and 7.5% acetic acid.

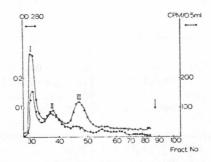

FIGURE 2: Sephadex G-100 gel filtration of the 100,000g supernatant fraction of the skin homogenate. The column was 2.5 × 140 cm, and 7.5 ml fractions were collected. The buffer was the same as for Figure 1, but without the β-mercaptoethanol. The mice had been treated with 1,2,5,6-dibenzanthracene.

Before measurements were made the gels were allowed to swell in 7.5% acetic acid. The system was standardized with proteins of known molecular weight.

Isoelectric Focusing in Polyacrylamide Gels. The method described by Wrigley (1968) was used. The gels consisted of A–H$_2$O (1:3, v/v). Solution A contained 0.8 ml of catalyst solution, 3.0 ml of acrylamide solution, and 0.3 ml of carrier ampholytes (40%). The catalyst solution contained 1 ml of N,N,N',N'-tetramethylethylenediamine and 14 mg of ribo-flavin, and was made to 100 ml with H$_2$O. The acrylamide solution contained 0.8 g of N,N'-methylenebisacrylamide and 30 g of acrylamide, and was made to 100 ml with H$_2$O. If the protein sample was mixed in the gels, 1 ml of gel mixture was used per tube (4 × 120 mm). If the sample was not mixed in the gel, 0.8 ml of gel mixture was used per tube. In the latter case the sample was put on top of the gel in 0.1 ml of 10% sucrose, on top of which 0.3 ml of 5% sucrose solution containing 1% carrier ampholytes was layered. The electrophoresis was carried out overnight in the cold room at 250 V; the last 1 or 2 hr were at 350 V. The gels were fixed and washed in 10% trichloroacetic acid, stained with coomassie brilliant blue in 10% trichloroacetic acid, and destained in 40% ethanol. Before measurements were made the gels were allowed to swell in 10% trichloroacetic acid.

For determination of the radioactivity the gels were cut into 1-mm slices with a gel slicer (Model 3015 Diversified Scientific Instruments, Inc.). The slices were then treated as described under measurements of radioactivity.

179

Results

Several extraction conditions for the mouse skin soluble proteins have been used during the years this work has been carried out. The most convenient method involves extraction with the same buffer (described in Materials and Methods) that is used for the subsequent column procedures. The homogenate thus extracted was centrifuged at 100,000g for 1 hr, and the supernatant fraction was passed through a Sephadex G-25 column. The high molecular weight fraction contained 25–30% of the OD_{280} units and radioactivity; the latter represents about 0.05% of the original amount of radioactivity applied to the skin as 1,2,5,6-dibenzanthracene-t. In the low molecular weight fraction, 90% of the label was accounted for as tritiated water, indicating that considerable

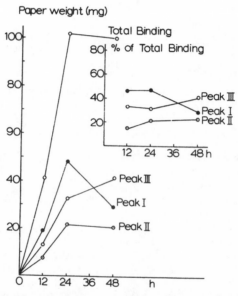

FIGURE 3: Time dependence of the binding of 1,2,5,6-dibenzanthracene-t to different high molecular weight fractions. At the indicated time after application, the 100,000g supernatant fraction was fractionated on Sephadex G-100 as shown in Figure 2; the radioactivity was determined in the individual fractions, and the results were graphed and expressed as the weight of the graph paper to give the integrated radioactivity.

exchange had occurred. However, this exchange could not account for the radioactivity in the h protein because of the large dilution, the nonuniform distribution among the various

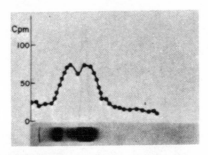

FIGURE 4: Polyacrylamide gel disc electrophoresis of the *h* protein fraction after Sephadex G-100 fractionation of the DEAE-cellulose eluate of proteins extracted from mice treated with 1,2,5,6-DBA. The graph shows the distribution of the radioactivity.

soluble proteins, and current studies in the laboratory on the structure of the protein-bound hydrocarbon derivatives.

The least acidic protein fraction was obtained by chromatography on DEAE-cellulose, by which Moore and Lee (1960) had separated the basic proteins of rat liver. They used an initial buffer of 0.005 M Tris–phosphate (pH 8.0) and subsequently a gradient to 0.5 M sodium phosphate, pH 6.5. We adopted a two-step elution first with 0.01 M Tris-HCl (pH 8.0) containing 0.01 M NaCl followed by 0.05 M sodium phosphate (pH 6.5) containing 1 M NaCl. The protein fraction (8–10%) that was not retained by the column, had a specific activity 2–2.5-fold higher than that from the Sephadex G-25. The protein fraction eluted with the second buffer had about a 5-fold lower specific activity than the first fraction.

When Sephadex G-100 gel filtration was carried out on the first fraction from the DEAE-cellulose column, a single symmetrical peak of radioactivity was obtained as shown in Figure 1 (MCA-treated mice) and as also reported by Umeda *et al.* (1968). With the 0.01 M Tris-HCl buffer (pH 8.0) containing 0.01 M NaCl, the recovery of radioactivity from the column was rather low (40–50%). The addition of 0.005 M β-mercaptoethanol increased the total recovery to 70–75%. A comparison of the elution volume of this radioactive peak from Sephadex G-100 with those of bovine serum albumin and horse heart cytochrome *c* gave, by the method of Andrews (1964), a molecular weight of about 40,000 for the *h* protein. When the second fraction eluted from the DEAE-cellulose column was run on a Sephadex G-100 column, nearly all the radioactivity was associated with molecules of a molecular weight greater than 40,000.

181

The Sephadex G-100 column was used directly to test the unfractionated skin supernatant fraction for the time course of the binding of 1,2,5,6-DBA. As shown in Figure 2, there were three peaks of high molecular weight with bound radioactivity, well separated from the small molecules. In agreement with the results of Abell and Heidelberger (1962), the maximum specific activity was found 24–48 hr after application of the hydrocarbons as shown in Figure 3. The mouse skin *h* protein fraction is found in the third peak of Figure 2, which shows an increasing amount of radioactivity until 48 hr.

The single sharp and symmetrical radioactive peak obtained on Sephadex G-100 fractionation of the DEAE-cellulose eluate from mice treated with MCA (Figure 1) suggested that at this stage of purification we might have had one protein to which the radioactive hydrocarbon was bound together with other nonradioactive proteins. However, polyacrylamide electrophoresis never resulted in a sharp radioactive peak (Figure 4) and the fact that chromatography of the skin *h* protein after Sephadex G-100 fractionation on CM-cellulose showed a radioactive pattern definitely not consistent with one radioactive protein (Figure 5), demonstrated that we had not yet achieved purity.

Further proof for the presence of more than one labeled protein in the radioactive *h* protein fraction after the Sephadex G-100 column came from a comparison, using these methods, of the binding of MCA, 1,2,5,6-DBA, and its non- (or very weakly) carcinogenic isomer, 1,2,3,4-DBA to the *h* protein fraction.

The results summarized in Table I show that MCA was bound to a greater extent than the two dibenzanthracenes at

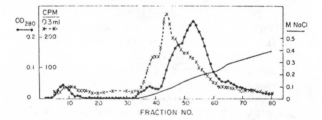

FIGURE 5: Carboxymethylcellulose chromatography of the same protein sample described for Figure 4. The column was 1.8 × 3.4 cm, and the buffer was 0.01 M Na_2HPO_4 plus 0.01 M acetic acid (pH 5.5) to which an NaCl gradient was added. Fractions of 1 ml were collected.

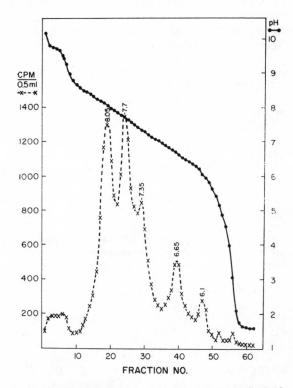

FIGURE 6: Isoelectric focusing in a column of the *h* protein obtained after the usual purification procedure following Sephadex G-100 fractionation. A pH gradient of 6–9 was used, and after 3 days of isoelectric focusing, fractions of 36 drops were collected. The radioactivity and the pH are graphed. The proteins were extracted from mice that had been treated with 1,2,5,6-dibenzanthracene-*t*.

all stages of purification except the initial Sephadex G-25 column. Although there was some radioactivity from 1,2,3,4-DBA in the least acidic fraction (DEAE-cellulose breakthrough peak), starch gel electrophoresis of this fraction derived from the skins treated with both hydrocarbons confirmed the earlier results (Abell and Heidelberger, 1962) of a labeled band in the basic protein region that was much

TABLE I: Binding of Hydrocarbons to the Protein Fractions at Different Stages of Purification.

	$\mu\mu$mol of Hydrocarbon/ OD_{280}		
Hydrocarbon	MCA[a]	1,2,5,6-DBA[b]	1,2,3,4-DBA[c]
Sephadex G-25 high molecular weight fraction	21	25	20
DEAE-cellulose breakthrough peak	68	46	34
Sephadex G-100 radioactive fraction	494	233	140

[a] Average of 6 experiments, 1200 mice. [b] Average of 12 experiments, 1100 mice. [c] Average of 3 experiments, 300 mice.

more radioactive in the case of the carcinogenic 1,2,5,6-DBA. However, when the partially purified proteins were compared on Sephadex G-100 columns, both were eluted in the same region. The only difference was an additional small peak (occurring in the region of fraction 45 in Figure 1), just before the main peak, that contained about 15% of the label from 1,2,3,4-DBA.

Further separation and purification of the radioactive proteins in the Sephadex G-100 fraction was carried out by the isoelectric focusing method developed by Vesterberg and Svensson (1966), which has excellent resolving capability. The results obtained by this technic with a pH gradient from 6 to 9 on the proteins derived from 1,2,5,6-DBA, 1,2,3,4-DBA, and MCA are shown in Figures 6–8. Several replicate experiments were carried out with the proteins derived from application of each hydrocarbon with excellent reproducibility. These isoelectric focusing fractionations show clearly that the single symmetrical radioactive peak eluted from the Sephadex G-100 column contains more than one labeled protein. Furthermore, they show that with both carcinogens there was a sharp radioactive peak at pH 8.05 that was not found with 1,2,3,4-DBA. Therefore, by definition, this peak is the *h* protein from mouse skin.

It was rather difficult to obtain an accurate picture of the position of the nonradioactive proteins in the isoelectric focusing procedure because our samples contained very small amounts of proteins (6–8 OD_{280} units from 100 mice) and the ampholytes also absorb to some extent at 280 mμ,

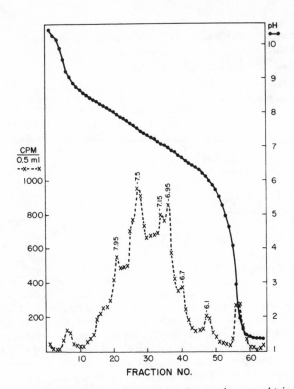

FIGURE 7: Same as Figure 6, except that the proteins were obtained from mice treated with 1,2,3,4-dibenzanthracene-*t*.

although considerably less than at 260 mμ. This fact also prevented us from obtaining accurate specific activities in all cases. However, in the experiment described in Table II,

185

	% Radio-activity in h Protein Fraction	Increase in Sp Act. (-fold)	Total Purificn[a] (-fold)
Sephadex G-25 high molecular weight fraction			0
DEAE-cellulose breakthrough peak	25	3	12
Sephadex G-100 fraction	100	7	84
Isoelectric focusing fraction pH 8.05[b]	30	2	560

[a] Since the h protein is only one of many radioactive proteins in the original extract, its increase in specific activity is not enough to indicate purification. In addition, it is necessary to determine on a given column or procedure, how much of the total radioactivity is present as h protein and divide the purity calculated from the specific activity by that value. In other words, the purification of the radioactive h protein involves its separation and removal from other radioactive proteins. [b] Since the protein concentration could not be determined in the presence of ampholytes by OD_{230} measurements, the tubes in this experiment were individually dialyzed extensively against water, and the protein concentration was then determined by OD_{280} values.

individual tubes were dialyzed and their protein contents were determined by OD_{280} measurements. This revealed that 30% of the radioactivity was present in the h protein fraction at pH 8.05 obtained from mice treated with MCA, and corresponds to a purification of 560-fold. In this pH 8.05

fraction, the actual specific activity was 240×10^3 dpm/OD$_{280}$, corresponding to 1090 $\mu\mu$mol of MCA/OD$_{280}$. Assuming a molecular weight of 40,000 for the protein, and that the bound hydrocarbon's specific activity was the same as that applied to the skin, 4-5% of the protein molecules in this fraction

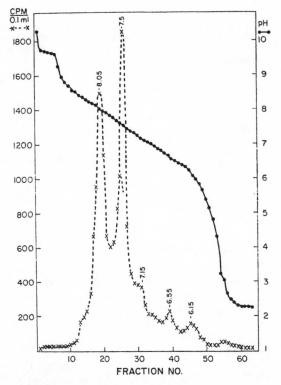

FIGURE 8: Same as Figure 6, except that the mice were treated with 3-methylcholanthrene-t.

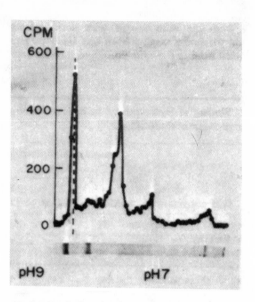

FIGURE 9: Isoelectric focusing in a polyacrylamide gel of the same protein fraction as described in Figure 8. Carrier ampholytes in the pH range of 7–9 were used. The sample was layered on the gel after polymerization.

would have hydrocarbons attached. This fraction contained about 4% of the radioactivity in the original protein extract.

In order to gain further information on the protein distribution in the eluate from Sephadex G-100, isoelectric focusing was carried out in polyacrylamide gels by the method of Wrigley (1968). The results of a typical experiment are shown in Figure 9, in which two peaks of radioactivity were found at essentially the same pH as in the isoelectric focusing column (Figure 8). The first peak at pH 8.05 coincides with a faintly stained band that is very close to a heavily stained protein band. The second radioactive peak at pH 7.5 was in the region of a very faintly stained band, and no radioactivity was associated with a second heavily stained protein band (Figure 9). The heavily stained band adjacent to the pH 8.05 peak was also found in the fraction isolated from the corresponding peak of the isoelectric focusing column, as revealed both by conventional electrophoresis and isoelectric focusing in polyacrylamide gels, probably because of some band spreading during the collection of fractions from the column.

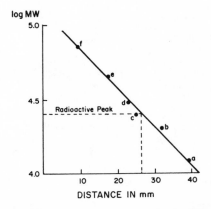

FIGURE 10: Standard curve for the sodium dodecyl sulfate, urea, and polyacrylamide gel system. The proteins used were (a) cytochrome c; (b) bromgrass mosaic virus; (c) elastase, (d) DNase I, (e) ovalbumin, and (f) transferrin.

At this stage, it appeared worthwhile to determine again the molecular weight of the h protein, which was found to be 40,000 on the original Sephadex G-100 column. After isoelectric focusing column purification of the protein derived from mice treated with MCA, the pH 8.05 peak contained so little protein that molecular weight determination on Sephadex G-100 was impossible. Therefore, we turned to polyacrylamide gel electrophoresis. When the molecular weight was determined by electrophoresis in gels of varying concentrations by the method of Hedrick and Smith (1968) a value of 40,000 was again found. Here, the gels contained one stained band

189

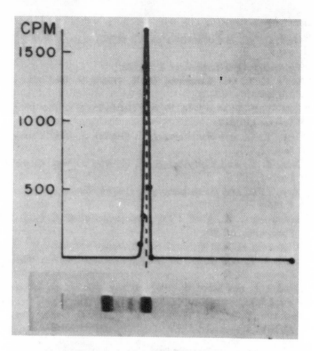

FIGURE 11: Sodium dodecyl sulfate polyacrylamide gel electrophoresis of the *h* protein fraction obtained from the pH 8.05 peak of the isoelectric focusing column. The mice had been treated with MCA.

and one sharp peak of radioactivity that coincided with the upper part of the stained band. We also resorted to polyacrylamide gel electrophoresis in the presence of sodium dodecyl sulfate and 8 M urea, according to the method devised by Shapiro *et al.* (1967). This method was calibrated with six purified proteins of known molecular weight (Figure 10), and a better standard curve was obtained than we had found with the method employing different gel concentrations. Electrophoresis in the sodium dodecyl sulfate–urea system of the *h* protein eluted from the pH 8.05 peak in the preparative electrofocusing column gave, as shown in Figure 11, a single very sharp radioactive peak at a molecular weight of 20,000 coinciding with one of two bands. The nonradioactive band corresponded to a molecular weight of 46,000. This result suggests that the *h* protein consists of two subunits of mol wt 20,000, together with a contaminating nonradioactive protein with a molecular weight of 46,000. Similar experiments with the *h* protein purified in the same way from the skin of mice treated with 1,2,5,6-DBA also demonstrated that it consists of two subunits of 20,000 molecular weight.

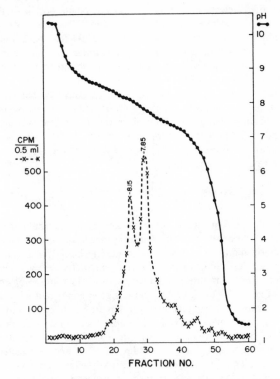

FIGURE 12: Isoelectric focusing on a column in a gradient of pH 7–9 of the same protein described in Figure 11.

Since the *h* protein obtained in the pH 8.05 peak from the electrofocusing column contained at least one nonradioactive protein contaminant of the single radioactive protein, attempts were made to purify it further by rerunning the peak on a second isoelectric focusing column, this time in a pH gradient of 7–9. Surprisingly, as shown in Figure 12, two peaks were obtained at pH 8.15 and 7.85. It seemed unlikely that this separation resulted from better resolution in this pH gradient. This was verified by the finding that when the *h* protein after Sephadex G-100 was run on an isoelectric focusing column in a pH gradient of 7–9 the distribution of radioactivity was

191

completely comparable with that found (Figures 6–8) at a pH gradient of 6–9. Furthermore, when the peak at pH 7.5 from the isoelectric focusing column was rerun, only a single labeled peak at the same pH was obtained. The two proteins obtained by reisoelectric focusing of the pH 8.05 peak were electrophoresed in gels of varying acrylamide concentrations, and the molecular weights of both were found to be about 40,000. This shows that the second isoelectric focusing procedure did not split the protein into the subunits that were produced by sodium dodecyl sulfate and urea. However, the splitting of the pH 8.05 peak into two proteins was also found in isoelectric focusing experiments in gels when the sample was present during the polymerization. Thus, the nature of this effect is unknown.

Discussion

In the present work we have accomplished the partial purification of the protein fraction from mouse skin to which carcinogenic hydrocarbons are covalently bound in a quantitative relationship to their carcinogenic activities; we have named this the mouse skin *h* protein, after the terminology of Sorof *et al.* (*cf.* 1967, 1969), who has been concerned with an apparently somewhat similar protein in rat liver to which hepatocarcinogenic amines are bound. Our purification procedure has involved successive fractionations on Sephadex G-25, DEAE-cellulose, Sephadex G-100, and isoelectric focusing. The final stage of this partial purification gives us a single radioactive protein with an isoelectric point of pH 8.05, contaminated with at least one other nonradioactive protein.

The degree of purification cannot be calculated in the same way in which enzyme purifications are, since in enzyme purifications there is usually only one given enzyme in an extract, whereas the *h* protein is only one of many radioactive proteins in the skin extract. Since radioactivity is our only measure of *h* protein, the degree of purification must be calculated so as to account for the removal from a given fraction of radioactive proteins other than the *h* protein, as explained in footnote *a* of Table II. In a typical experiment following application of MCA, the *h* protein in the pH 8.05 fraction from an isoelectric focusing column has been purified 560-fold (Table II) and represents a recovery of 4% of the radioactivity in the skin extract. This does not mean a 4% yield, since there are many other radioactive proteins in the extract.

We have demonstrated that the mouse skin *h* protein has a molecular weight of 40,000 and that it is made up of two subunits of 20,000 molecular weight. There appears to be some difference of opinion about the molecular weight of the corresponding protein obtained from rat liver. Sorof (1969) has reported a molecular weight of 60,000–80,000, determined by Sephadex G-200 chromatography, and Ketterer *et al.* (1967) found a molecular weight of 45,000 by Sephadex G-100 chromatography and sedimentation analysis. It is conceivable that the latter protein is a subunit of the former. If that is so, then the liver protein has twice the molecular weight of the mouse skin protein that we have been concerned with.

An interesting finding has been made by Freed and Sorof (1966, 1967) that an electrophoretic fraction of rat liver protein containing bound aminoazo dyes had the property of reversibly inhibiting the growth of cells. More recently Sorof *et al.* (1967) have shown that this growth inhibition is caused by arginase. We examined the mouse skin *h* protein fraction obtained after Sephadex G-100 fractionation, and found it to be devoid of arginase and growth inhibitory activities (Umeda *et al.*, 1968). Thus, the question of the involvement of arginase in chemical carcinogenesis remains open.

Why have we gone to the trouble to attempt to isolate and purify this problem? What is its role, if any, in chemical carcinogenesis? As described earlier (Abell and Heidelberger, 1962), there is an impressive correlation between the binding of hydrocarbons to the mouse skin *h* protein and the process of carcinogenesis. In fact, we believe that this correlation is better with respect to carcinogenesis than is the correlation of the covalent binding to mouse skin DNA (Goshman and Heidelberger, 1967). However, such correlations certainly do not constitute proof. Nevertheless, they justify the present work. Since it now seems to be clear that in almost all cases that have been properly studied chemical carcinogens are covalently bound to DNA, RNA, and protein, it is very difficult to determine conclusively which (if any) of these interactions is of causal significance in carcinogenesis. To our knowledge, no such determination has been made with any chemical carcinogen. Pitot and Heidelberger (1963) have offered a theory as to how the binding of a carcinogenic hydrocarbon to the *h* protein could give rise to a perpetuated change.

The recent development in our laboratory of a quantitative system for obtaining carcinogenesis *in vitro* of cells derived from C3H mouse prostate with carcinogenic hydrocarbons (Chen and Heidelberger, 1969a–c) provides the opportunity to test the possible role of the mouse skin *h* protein in the carcinogenic process.

References

Abell, C. W., and Heidelberger, C. (1962), *Cancer Res. 22*, 931.

Andrews, P. (1964), *Biochem. J. 91*, 222.

Barry, E. J., and Gutmann, H. R. (1966), *J. Biol. Chem. 241*, 4600.

Blatt, W. F., Feinberg, M. P., and Hopfenberg, H. B. (1965), *Science 150*, 224.

Chen, T. T., and Heidelberger, C. (1969a), *J. Natl. Cancer Inst. 42*, 903.

Chen, T. T., and Heidelberger, C. (1969b), *J. Natl. Cancer Inst. 42*, 915.

Chen, T. T., and Heidelberger, C. (1969c), *Intern. J. Cancer 4*, 166.

Davenport, G. R., Abell, C. W., and Heidelberger, C. (1961), *Cancer Res. 21*, 599.

Determann, H., and Walter, I. (1968), *Nature 219*, 604.

Freed, J. J., and Sorof, S. (1966), *Biochem. Biophys. Res. Commun. 22*, 1.

Freed, J. J., and Sorof, S. (1967), *Wistar. Inst. Symp. Monograph 7*, 15.

Goshman, L. M., and Heidelberger, C. (1967), *Cancer Res. 27*, 1678.

Hedrick, J. L., and Smith, A. J. (1968), *Arch. Biochem. Biophys. 126*, 155.

Heidelberger, C., and Moldenhauer, M. G. (1956), *Cancer Res. 16*, 442.

Ketterer, B., Ross-Mansell, P., and Whitehead, J. K. (1967), *Biochem. J. 103*, 316.

Miller, E. C. (1951), *Cancer Res. 11*, 100.

Moore, B. W., and Lee, R. H. (1960), *J. Biol. Chem. 235*, 1359.

Pitot, H. C., and Heidelberger, C. (1963), *Cancer Res. 23*, 1694.

Shapiro, A. L., Vinuela, E., and Maizel, J. V. (1967), *Biochem. Biophys. Res. Commun. 28*, 815.

Sorof, S. (1969), *Jerusalem Symp. Quantum Chem. Biochem. 1*, 208.

Sorof, S., Young, E. M., Luongo, L., Kish, V. M., and Freed, J. J. (1967), *Wistar Inst. Symp. Monograph 7*, 25.

Sorof, S., Young, E. M., McCue, M. M., and Fetterman, P. L. (1963), *Cancer Res. 23*, 864.

Umeda, M., Diringer, H., and Heidelberger, C. (1968), *Israel J. Med. Sci. 4*, 1216.

Vesterberg, O., and Svensson, H. (1966), *Acta Chem. Scand. 20*, 820.

Wiest, W. G., and Heidelberger, C. (1953), *Cancer Res. 13*,

250.
Wrigley, C. (1968), *Sci. Tools 15*, 17.
Young, R. W., and Fulhorst, H. W. (1965), *Anal. Biochem.*
  11, 389.

Coding and Conformational Properties of Oligonucleotides Modified with the Carcinogen N-2-Acetylaminofluorene*

Dezider Grunberger, James H. Nelson, Charles R. Cantor, and I. Bernard Weinstein

Introduction. N-2-Acetylaminofluorene (AAF) is a potent hepatic carcinogen which, after metabolic activation, binds to liver RNA, DNA, and protein when administered in vivo.[1-7] Miller et al.[5] have demonstrated that a synthetically prepared ester, N-acetoxy-2-acetylaminofluorene (N-acetoxy AAF), complexes directly with RNA and DNA at neutral pH in vitro. Hydrolysis of liver RNA obtained from rats given AAF in vivo, or RNA reacted with N-acetoxy-AAF in vitro, indicates that the major nucleoside derivative is 8-(N-2-fluorenylacetamido) guanosine.[6] There is evidence that the attachment of AAF to DNA inhibits its template activity for RNA synthesis,[8] inhibits the transforming activity of B. subtilis DNA,[9] and is mutagenic.[9, 10] The attachment of AAF to tRNA produces specific modifications in amino acid acceptance capacity and codon recognition.[11]

The present studies were undertaken to explore the mechanism by which attachment of AAF residues to nucleic acids might distort their structure and thereby their biological activity. In contrast to certain other types of chemical modifications, the presence of an AAF residue on the 8 position of guanosine would not be expected to directly interfere with hydrogen bonding and base pairing.[6, 12] Previous data obtained with AAF-modified tRNA led to the suggestion that the observed changes in biologic activity might be caused by a conformational change in the nucleic acid.[11] We have now simplified the analysis of this problem by examining the functional properties of certain oligonucleotides, previously modified with N-acetoxy-AAF, in a ribosomal binding assay, and also obtained information on the conformation of these oligonucleotides by examining their circular dichroism spectra.

Materials and Methods. **Materials:** N-Acetoxy-AAF was generously supplied by Dr. James Miller of the University of Wisconsin. Poly (U,G) (3:1) and ApApG (AAG) were products of Miles Laboratories. GpUpU (GUU) and GpU were synthesized as previously described.[13] ApG, GpA, and UpG were purchased from Sigma Chemical Co. *E. coli* tRNA was purchased from General Biochemicals. Uniformly labeled [14C] amino acids, obtained from Schwarz BioResearch, had the following specific activities in mCi/mmole: valine (142), phenylalanine (510), and lysine (208). Ribonuclease T₂ was obtained from Sankyo, Tokyo.

Aminoacylation of tRNA and ribosomal binding assay: *E. coli* aminoacyl-tRNA synthetase was prepared from the 105,000 g supernatant fraction by chromatography on a DEAE-cellulose column. The material which eluted with 0.25 M NaCl in Tris-HCl (pH 7.5) was used as the enzyme fraction. The reaction mixture for preparing [14C]aminoacyl-tRNA's contained in a total volume of 1 ml: 0.01 M Tris-HCl (pH 7.5), 0.01 M MgCl₂, 0.01 M KCl, 0.002 M ATP, 20–100 A_{260} units of tRNA, and 1 mg of aminoacyl-tRNA synthetase. The reaction mixture was incubated at 37°C for 10 min, extracted with phenol, and the [14C]aminoacyl-tRNA precipitated with ethanol and stored at −20°C.

Ribosomes were prepared from *E. coli* B (General Biochemicals) as described.[14] The binding assay was that of Nirenberg and Leder[15] and is described in detail in Table 1.

TABLE 1. *The effect of AAF modification of oligo- and polynucleotides upon their stimulation of [14C]aminoacyl-tRNA binding to ribosomes.*

Polynucleotide (0.1 A_{260} nm)	[14C]aminoacyl-tRNA Bound					
	Valyl- (12.2 pmol)		Lysyl- (17 pmol)		Phenylalanyl- (6.5 pmole)	
	pmole	Δpmole	pmole	Δpmole	pmole	Δpmole
None	0.35	...	0.67	...	0.32	...
GUU	1.70	1.35	...	...	...	...
AAF-GUU	0.36	0.01	...	...	...	...
AAG	...	...	1.46	0.79	...	...
AAG-AAF	...	...	0.68	0.01	...	...
Poly (U,G)	5.87	5.52	...	...	4.20	3.88
Poly (U,G)-AAF	3.44	3.09	...	...	4.22	3.90

The incubation mixture (0.05 ml) contained 0.10 M Tris-acetate (pH 7.2), 0.05 M KCl, 0.03 M magnesium acetate, and 2–2.5 A_{260} units of *E. coli* ribosomes. [14C]aminoacyl-tRNA, trinucleotides, and polymers were added as specified in the table. Incubation was performed at 24°C for 20 min, and samples processed and counted as described.[15]

Reaction of N-acetoxy-AAF with oligonucleotides and poly (U,G): N-acetoxy-AAF (5 × 10⁻³ M) was reacted at 37°C for 3 hr with 10–50 A_{260} units of oligonucleotides in 1 ml of 0.1 M Tris-HCl pH 7.2 and 33% ethanol, under nitrogen. The free drug was then extracted from the reaction mixture twice with ethyl ether. Oligonucleotides modified with AAF were purified by paper chromatography (see below).

N-Acetoxy-AAF (17.5 × 10⁻³ M) was reacted at 37°C for 3 hr with 30 A_{260} units of poly (U,G) in 2 ml of 0.05 M citrate buffer (pH 7.0) and 33% ethanol, under nitrogen. The mixture was extracted twice with an equal volume of ethyl ether and the modified polymer precipitated with ethanol.

Chromatography and base composition: Oligonucleotides containing AAF were separated from the unreacted materials by paper chromatography on Whatman 3MM with a mixture of n-butanol, acetic acid, water (5:2:3, v/v/v). R_f values were; GUU and AAG, 0.08; AAF-GUU and AAG-AAF, 0.38: UpG, ApG, and GpA, 0.17; and the AAF containing dinucleoside phosphates, 0.64. Under ultraviolet light, the compounds containing AAF had a blue fluorescence. Compounds were eluted with water and their spectra determined.

The base composition of oligonucleotides and polymers was determined by digestion of 1 to 2 A_{260} units of sample with 2 units of ribonuclease T_2 in 0.05 ml of 0.05 M sodium acetate (pH 4.65) for 18 hr at 37°C. The products were separated by two-dimensional thin-layer chromatography on 10 × 10 cm MN 300 cellulose plates (Brinkman Instruments). The solvents were: (a) isobutyric acid-0.5 M NH₄OH (5:3, v/v) for the first dimension and (b) isopropanol-conc HCl-H₂O (7:1.5:1.5, v/v/v) for the second dimension. The AAF containing guanosine residue had a rapid mobility in both solvents and was readily detected by its blue-green fluorescence under ultraviolet light.

Spectral methods: Ultraviolet absorption spectra were determined with a Beckman DBG spectrophotometer. Circular dichroism spectra were recorded on a Cary 60 spectropolarimeter equipped with a Cary model 6001 circular dichroism accessory. Oligonucleotide samples for circular dichroism spectra were studied at approximately 5 × 10⁻⁵ M in 0.005 M phosphate buffer (pH 6.9) and 0.05 M NaClO₄. Extinction coefficients of oligonucleotides were calculated from the extinction coefficients of the respective monomer constituents, with appropriate correction for hypochromic effects.[16] An extinction coefficient at 260 nm of 29 × 10³ was assumed for AAF-guanosine.[6] Hypochromic effects caused by AAF were ignored.

Results. Binding of AAF to GUU, AAG, and poly (U,G): Figure 1 compares the absorption spectra of GUU, which had been previously reacted with N-acetoxy-AAF and purified by paper chromatography (AAF-GUU), to that of a control sample of GUU. The modified material showed a shift in absorption maximum from 257 to 265 mμ and a shoulder at 300–310 mμ, which was not seen with GUU. Similar changes in the absorption spectra of nucleic acids modified with N-acetoxy-AAF have been previously described[5, 6, 11] and reflect the presence of the bound AAF. After ribonuclease T_2 digestion and thin-layer chromatography, Up, U, and Gp-AAF, but no Gp, were detected. In the modified triplet, therefore, all of the G residues were substituted with AAF. The absorption spectrum of AAG modified with AAF also revealed a shift in absorption maximum to a higher wavelength and the appearance of a shoulder at 300–310 mμ.

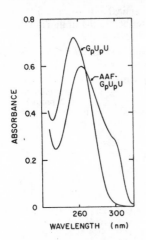

FIG. 1.—Ultraviolet absorption spectra of GUU and AAF-GUU.

Base composition analysis of the modified AAG also indicated complete substitution of guanosine residues with AAF.

When poly (U,G) (3:1) was reacted with N-acetoxy-AAF and repurified (see *Materials and Methods*), changes in the absorption spectrum similar to those described above were seen. Digestion with ribonuclease T_2 and base composition analysis indicated that 40% of the guanosine residues were modified by AAF. Additional studies indicated that the degree of modification was dependent on the concentration of N-acetoxy-AAF in the reaction mixture.

Codon recognition: Table 1 compares the abilities of GUU and AAF-GUU to stimulate binding of [¹⁴C]valyl-tRNA to ribosomes. Whereas [¹⁴C]valyl-tRNA recognized the valine codon GUU, there was no response of [¹⁴C]valyl-tRNA to the AAF-containing triplet.   Modification of G by AAF also completely inhibited the function of AAG in ribosomal binding of [¹⁴C]lysyl-tRNA (Table 1). It is apparent, therefore, that modification of the G residue with AAF, in either the 5'- or 3'-end of a triplet, inactivates codon recognition.

In view of the results obtained with triplets, we also examined the effect of AAF modification on the ability of poly (U,G) to stimulate ribosomal binding of phenylalanyl- and valyl-tRNA's.   Table 1 indicates that the binding of [¹⁴C]-valyl-tRNA to ribosomes in the presence of poly (U,G)-AAF was decreased by approximately 40% of that obtained with the same concentration of unmodified poly (U,G).   This decrease corresponds to the extent of G modification by AAF revealed from base composition data (see above).   On the other hand, the stimulation of ribosomal binding of [¹⁴C]phenylalanyl-tRNA was not impaired by AAF modification, indicating that the UUU sequences contained within the same polymer remain functional and, therefore, AAF does not impair ribosomal binding of the polymer.

Circular dichroism spectra of oligomers: The conformational properties of AAF-modified nucleic acid derivatives was examined by circular dichroism spectra.   Figures 2 and 3 present the molar ellipticity, $[\theta]$, as a function of wavelength for the compounds: GMP, ApG, GpA, UpG, GUU, and their corresponding AAF-substituted derivatives.   One must be cautious in interpreting these circular dichroism spectra, because it is difficult to distinguish between: (1) optical activity induced in AAF because of its attachment to a guanosine residue, or because of interaction of AAF with other chromophores of the oligonucleotide, and (2) optical activity resulting from changes in conformation of the nucleoside

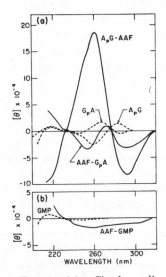

Fig. 2.—(a) Circular dichroism curves of ApG; GpA, ApG-AAF, and AAF-GpA.
(b) Circular dichroism curves of GMP and AAF-GMP.

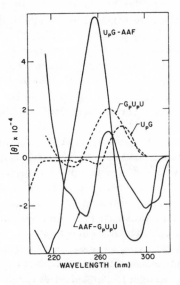

Fig. 3.—Circular dichroism curves of UpG, GpUpU, UpG-AAF, and AAF-GpUpU.

residues. It was, therefore, necessary to examine the circular dichroism spectrum of AAF-substituted GMP (AAF-GMP). Figure 2b indicates that AAF substitution does alter the circular dichroism spectral characteristics of GMP. The dichroism of GMP is fairly weak, and there is little optical activity observed at wavelengths greater than 270 nm. AAF-GMP, however, has a relatively strong negative dichroism in the spectral region of 240–310 nm. Since AAF has a high extinction coefficient in this region, it is likely that the strong dichroism of AAF-GMP at these wavelengths results from optical activity induced in AAF by covalent attachment to guanosine. The circular dichroism spectrum of AAF-GMP is also much different from that of guanosine at lower wavelengths (200–240 nm).

Figure 2a shows that the spectra of unsubstituted ApG and GpA are quite unlike each other. These differences, which may be attributed to the difference in the interactions of the transition moments of the base chromophores in the respective base-stacked sequence isomers,[17] illustrate the effect of changes in the relative conformation of the two bases on the circular dichroism spectra. Of particular interest are the striking changes in the spectra of ApG and GpA produced by AAF substitution (Fig. 2a). Somewhat similar changes were also observed with UpG and GUU (Fig. 3). These large spectral changes are not simply the result of covalent bonding of AAF to guanosine residues because the differences between the spectra of each oligonucleotide and its derivative are much greater than the corresponding difference between guanosine and AAF-GMP. This observation, together with the fact that the dichroism of the AAF-modified oligonucleotides is very strong at wavelengths greater than 290 nm, where only the AAF moiety absorbs significantly, indicates that AAF interacts with the base adjacent to the substituted guanine. The spectrum of ApG-AAF is particularly striking (Fig. 2). The strength of the circular dichroism observed for this substituted dinucleotide is an order of magnitude greater than that observed for either unsubstituted oligonucleotides or the substituted monomer. Although the dichroism of UpG-AAF is also unusually strong (Fig. 3) it is only about a third that of ApG-AAF in the region of the most intense circular dichroism band. The spectacularly large bands in ApG-AAF probably arise from a strong interaction of AAF with the adjacent adenine residue (see *Discussion*). Although the spectra of ApG-AAF and AAF-GpA are substantially different, those of ApG-AAF and UpG-AAG are qualitatively quite similar. The same observation is also true for the spectra of AAF-GpA and AAF-GUU. Apparently AAF determines the basic spectral characteristics of the substituted oligonucleotides, and the quality of the alteration is largely dependent on whether the substituted guanosine is at the 5'- or the 3'-end of the oligomer.

Discussion: Although it is not possible at the present time to determine which conformation most closely approximates the average preferred configuration of the modified oligonucleotides, it is evident that the binding of AAF does introduce important conformational changes in these molecules. A study of molecular models of AAF-modified dinucleoside phosphates suggests that the most probable conformational change is a rotation of the modified guanosine about the glycosidic bond, followed by stacking of AAF with the base

200

adjacent to this guanine. This seems plausible for two reasons: Firstly, attachment of AAF to the 8 position of guanine is sterically hindered if the guanosine remains in the normal "anti" conformation with torsion angle values of ϕCN $\sim$ $-30°$C.[18] However, rotation about the glycosidic bond to torsional angles ϕCN $\sim$ $+50°$ to $150°$ will relieve this hindrance (see Fig. 4). Secondly, the circular dichroism data suggest that AAF strongly interacts with the neighboring base, presumably because the large hydrocarbon tends to stack with nonpolar bases. This would disrupt the normal base stacking between guanine and its adjacent base. Similar conformational

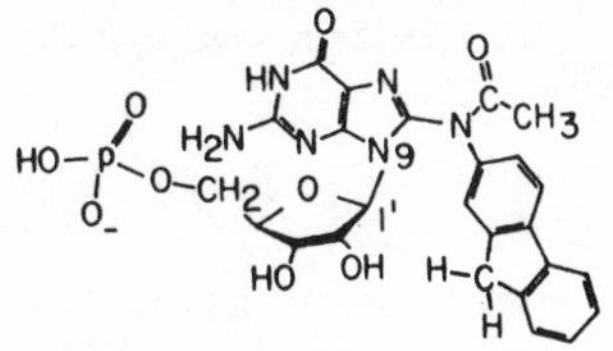

FIG. 4.—Schematic representation of AAF-GMP. In contrast to the normal configuration of GMP, the guanine base has been rotated approximately 180° about the N(9)-C(1') bond to minimize steric hindrance with the bulky AAF residue.

changes at sites of AAF substitution in coding triplets would make it difficult for the normal hydrogen-bonding sites of the respective bases along the nucleotide chain to become sufficiently aligned, with respect to orientation and distance, to effect binding to complementary sites on the anticodon of tRNA. A similar effect would also be expected for higher molecular weight polynucleotides. The present data do not exclude other types of conformational alterations induced by AAF. Circular dichroism spectra, as well as nuclear magnetic resonance studies, on the conformations of additional AAF-modified oligonucleotides and polynucleotides are currently in progress.

The relationship of these findings to the carcinogenic activity of AAF is not known. Conformational changes produced by AAF could profoundly alter the biologic properties of both cellular RNA and DNA. The relative susceptibility of specific guanosine residues to AAF modification, as well as effects of base sequence on the type of conformational distortion which occurs, might contribute to the biologic specificity of this carcinogen. If attack on the DNA, with subsequent somatic mutation, is the critical event, than a conformational change would be more likely to produce small deletions rather than single base changes during DNA replication (see ref. 9 for a summary of conflicting data on this point). A conformational change in specific regions of the DNA might also impair the transcription of certain genetic loci. With respect to RNA, an AAF-induced conformational change in tRNA would explain the previously observed inhibitions of tRNA aminoacylation and codon recognition.[11] The present results indicate that if AAF binds to mRNA's *in vivo*, it would also inhibit their function in protein synthesis. These, as well as additional effects on cellular RNA's, might lead to rather widespread disturbances in the translation apparatus with secondary consequences with respect to cell differentiation, regulation, and autonomy.[19]

We are pleased to acknowledge the valuable technical assistance of Miss Gloria Carvajal.

Abbreviations: A, adenosine; G, guanosine; U, uridine; C, cytidine; AAF, *N*-2-acetylaminofluorene; tRNA, transfer RNA. For oligonucleotides of specific structure, internal phosphodiesters (3'-5') between nucleosides are indicated as in ApG for adenosine-guanosine monophosphate. Poly (U,G) (3:1) designates a random copolymer of uridylic and guanylic acids at a ratio of 3:1.

* This research was supported by grant CA-02332 and GM-14825 from the U.S. Public Health Service.

[1] Marroquin, F., and E. Farber, *Cancer Res.*, **25**, 1262 (1965).
[2] Henshaw, E. C., and H. H. Hiatt, *Proc. Amer. Assoc. Canc. Res.*, **4**, 27 (1963).
[3] Kriek, E., *Biochim. Biophys. Acta*, **161**, 273 (1968).
[4] Irving, C. C., R. A. Veazey, and R. F. Williard, *Cancer Res.*, **27**, 720 (1967).
[5] Miller, E. C., V. Juhl, and J. A. Miller, *Science*, **153**, 1125 (1966).
[6] Kriek, E., J. A. Miller, V. Juhl, and E. C. Miller, *Biochemistry*, **6**, 177 (1967).
[7] Agarwal, M. K., and I. B. Weinstein, *Biochemistry*, **9**, 503 (1970).
[8] Troll, W., S. Bellman, E. Berkowitz, Z. F. Chmielewicz, J. L. Ambrus, and T. J. Bardos, *Biochim. Biophys. Acta*, **157**, 16 (1968).
[9] Maher, V. M., E. C. Miller, J. A. Miller, and W. Szybalski, *Mol. Pharmacol.*, **4**, 411 (1968).
[10] Troll, W., *Cancer Res.*, **28**, 1870 (1968).
[11] Fink, L. M., S. Nishimura, and I. B. Weinstein, *Biochemistry*, **9**, 496 (1970).
[12] Crick, F. H. C., *J. Mol. Biol.*, **19**, 548 (1966).
[13] Grunberger, D., A. Holý, and F. Šorm, *Collection Czech. Chem. Commun.*, **33**, 286 (1968).
[14] Grunberger, D., L. Meissner, A. Holý, and F. Šorm, *Collection Czech. Chem. Commun.*, **32**, 2625 (1967).
[15] Nirenberg, M., and P. Leder, *Science*, **145**, 1399 (1964).
[16] Cantor, C. R., and I. Tinoco, Jr., *J. Mol. Biol.*, **13**, 64 (1965).
[17] Warshaw, M. M., and C. R. Cantor, *Biopolymers*, in press.
[18] For a definition of these angles see Donohue, J., and K. N. Trueblood, *J. Mol. Biol.*, **2**, 353 (1960).
[19] Weinstein, I. B., *Cancer Res.*, **28**, 1871 (1968).

KEY-WORD TITLE INDEX

AUTHOR INDEX

204